ORTHOPEDIC NAVIGATOR
An Orthopedic Guide for Postgraduates

ORTHOPEDIC NAVIGATOR
An Orthopedic Guide for Postgraduates

Editors

Jacob Ipe
MBBS Dip (Ortho) DNB (Ortho)
Consultant
Department of Orthopedics
Sapthagiri Medical College
Bengaluru, Karnataka, India

Febin Ahamed PI
MBBS MS (Ortho)
Fellow in Hand and Microvascular
Reconstruction Surgery
Department of Plastic, Hand and
Microvascular Reconstruction Surgery
Ganga Hospital
Coimbatore, Tamil Nadu, India

Jacob Eapen
MBBS MS (Ortho) DNB (Ortho)
Fellow in Arthroplasty (Depuy)
Fellow in Hand and Microvascular
Reconstruction Surgery
Department of Plastic, Hand and
Microvascular Reconstruction Surgery
Ganga Hospital
Coimbatore, Tamil Nadu, India

Forewords

Edward L Nazareth
George Abraham
Rajesh Purushothaman

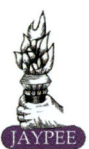

JAYPEE BROTHERS MEDICAL PUBLISHERS
The Health Sciences Publisher
New Delhi | London

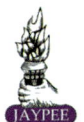 **Jaypee Brothers Medical Publishers (P) Ltd.**

Headquarters
Jaypee Brothers Medical Publishers (P) Ltd
EMCA House, 23/23-B
Ansari Road, Daryaganj
New Delhi 110 002, India
Landline: +91-11-23272143, +91-11-23272703
+91-11-23282021, +91-11-23245672
Email: jaypee@jaypeebrothers.com

Corporate Office
Jaypee Brothers Medical Publishers (P) Ltd
4838/24, Ansari Road, Daryaganj
New Delhi 110 002, India
Phone: +91-11-43574357
Fax: +91-11-43574314
Email: jaypee@jaypeebrothers.com

Overseas Office
J.P. Medical Ltd
83 Victoria Street, London
SW1H 0HW (UK)
Phone: +44 20 3170 8910
Fax: +44 (0)20 3008 6180
Email: info@jpmedpub.com

Website: www.jaypeebrothers.com
Website: www.jaypeedigital.com

© 2022, Jaypee Brothers Medical Publishers

The views and opinions expressed in this book are solely those of the original contributor(s)/author(s) and do not necessarily represent those of editor(s) of the book.

All rights reserved. No part of this publication may be reproduced, stored or transmitted in any form or by any means, electronic, mechanical, photocopying, recording or otherwise, without the prior permission in writing of the publishers.

All brand names and product names used in this book are trade names, service marks, trademarks or registered trademarks of their respective owners. The publisher is not associated with any product or vendor mentioned in this book.

Medical knowledge and practice change constantly. This book is designed to provide accurate, authoritative information about the subject matter in question. However, readers are advised to check the most current information available on procedures included and check information from the manufacturer of each product to be administered, to verify the recommended dose, formula, method and duration of administration, adverse effects and contraindications. It is the responsibility of the practitioner to take all appropriate safety precautions. Neither the publisher nor the author(s)/editor(s) assume any liability for any injury and/or damage to persons or property arising from or related to use of material in this book.

This book is sold on the understanding that the publisher is not engaged in providing professional medical services. If such advice or services are required, the services of a competent medical professional should be sought.

Every effort has been made where necessary to contact holders of copyright to obtain permission to reproduce copyright material. If any have been inadvertently overlooked, the publisher will be pleased to make the necessary arrangements at the first opportunity. The **CD/DVD-ROM** (if any) provided in the sealed envelope with this book is complimentary and free of cost. **Not meant for sale.**

Inquiries for bulk sales may be solicited at: jaypee@jaypeebrothers.com

Orthopedic Navigator: An Orthopedic Guide for Postgraduates

First Edition: **2022**

ISBN: 978-93-5465-203-5

Printed at: Sterling Graphics Pvt. Ltd.

Dedicated to

Parents and loved ones, teachers, friends, colleagues, and students

Our Beloved Teachers Who Taught us to Aim High

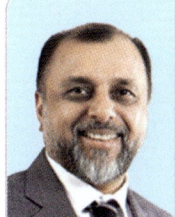

Sharan Shivraj Patil
MBBS MS (Ortho) MCh (Ortho) Liverpool FRCS (England)
Chairman
SPARSH Hospital
Bengaluru, Karnataka, India

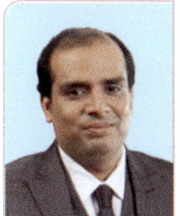

Ravikumar Mukartihal
MBBS Dip (Ortho) DNB (Ortho)
Senior Consultant
Department of Orthopedics
SPARSH Hospital
Bengaluru, Karnataka, India

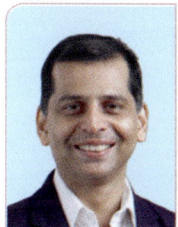

Gopalakrishnan ML
MBBS MS (Ortho) FNB (Hand and Microvascular Surgery)
Senior Consultant
Department of Orthopedics
Meitra Hospital
Calicut, Kerala, India

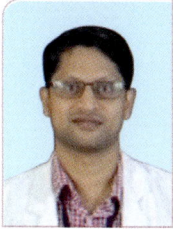

Prashanth Acharya
MBBS MS (Ortho) Fellow in Sports Medicine
Assistant Professor
Department of Orthopedics
Father Muller Medical College (FMMC)
Mangaluru, Karnataka, India

Our Beloved Teachers Who Taught us to Aim High

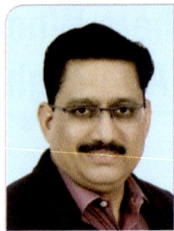

Niranjan Mallanaik
MBBS MS PhD (Ortho)
Senior Consultant
DNB Coordinator
Department of Orthopedics
Bangalore Baptist Hospital
Bengaluru, Karnataka, India

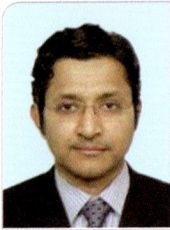

Vijay HD Kamath
MBBS MS (Ortho) FNBE (Spinal Surgery)
Fellow in Advanced Spinal Surgery (Honk Kong)
Head and Senior Consultant
Department of Orthopedics
Bangalore Baptist Hospital
Bengaluru, Karnataka, India

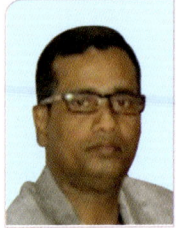

Birendra Kumar
MBBS MS (Ortho)
Senior Consultant
Department of Orthopedics
Bokaro General Hospital, SAIL/BSL
Jharkhand, India

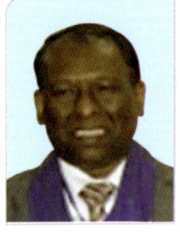

ND Kachhap
MBBS MS (Ortho)
Head and Senior Consultant
Department of Orthopedics
Bokaro General Hospital, SAIL/BSL
Jharkhand, India

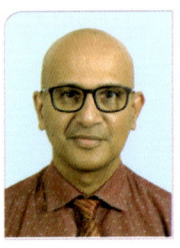

Anwar Marthya
MS (Ortho) Dip (Ortho) MRCSEd FRCS
Head
Department of Orthopedics
IQRAA International Hospital and
Research Centre
Calicut, Kerala, India

Foreword

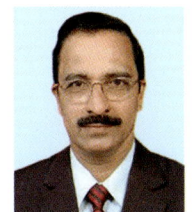

It is my pleasure and privilege to write this foreword to the book on basics of Orthopedics—classifications, radiological lines and diagnostic criteria which will help postgraduates in revising topics quickly. The included *Question Bank* will be a striking advantage to know what's expected in examinations.

I am greatly pleased with the authors of this book who were my postgraduate students at one time and immensely proud of this endeavor of theirs in joining together and coming out with this noble idea of sharing their preparations for the examinations with other students. When a postgraduate prepares for the orthopedic examinations, to remember these basic topics especially classifications is not easy. A ready reckoner will definitely come handy.

I congratulate the young and dynamic orthopedic surgeons—Dr Jacob Ipe, Dr Febin Ahamed PI, and Dr Jacob Eapen for this book. I wish them all the best and hope that they come out with more books in orthopedics in the future.

I wish every orthopedic postgraduate to keep a copy of this book with them and revise the topics as many times as possible so that their basics become strong.

Edward L Nazareth
MBBS Dip (Ortho) MS (Ortho)
Professor of Orthopedic Surgery
Father Muller Medical College
Mangaluru, Karnataka, India

Foreword

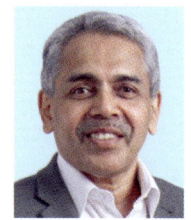

Orthopedic Navigator is a guide that will enable the postgraduate students when they are preparing for their examination. The comprehensive coverage of the subject and the included *Question Bank* will definitely help students to memorize what they have already read from exhaustive textbooks and stay sharp in their topics. The book will also be of great use to consultants who want to refresh the subject.

I congratulate the authors for undertaking such a herculean task and achieving a commendable result.

George Abraham
MS (Ortho) Dip (Ortho)
Fellow in Spine Surgery (Australia)
Chairman
Bone and Joint Care
Meitra Hospital
Calicut, Kerala, India

Foreword

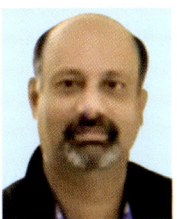

Orthopedics is a vast subject with rapidly expanding horizons. There are many classical textbooks in orthopedics, in addition there are many subspecialties, such as trauma, arthroplasty, arthroscopy, spine, hand, pediatric orthopedics, etc., with their own classic textbooks. While it is desirable and preferable to read all these original standard textbooks, it is practically impossible within the 3-year junior residency period.

It is very easy to get overwhelmed by the sheer quantity of information and knowledge available and get confused. In addition, the candidates often forget what they have read.

One of the solutions is to have books that act as navigators or cheat sheets that guide the candidates through the vast subject by providing a short summary, an overview or that highlights the salient points such as classifications, diagnostic criteria or various commonly used formulas. This book by the authors fulfills that purpose by providing the key learning points and condensed information about various common orthopedic conditions.

I am happy to recommend this book for the junior residents as a worthy addition to their backpacks and bookstands to expand their knowledge and to inspire them to search for more. I also recommend it to the senior consultants to gain some new points or to refresh their knowledge.

It is said that the best way to learn is to learn to teach the subject to someone else. The authors are an embodiment of this way. I wish them all the very best with this venture and in their future endeavors.

Rajesh Purushothaman
MBBS MS (Ortho)
Additional Professor of Orthopedics
Government Medical College
Calicut, Kerala, India

Preface

To be prepared is half victory. We all have been through the mental stress of preparing for examinations. This stress may also affect in a negative way during the examination preparation period.

Effective reading and utilizing time appropriately is what is needed when we face university examinations. Orthopedics is a vast subject with many standard textbooks to be followed, but during the examination period it may not be possible to revise from the various standard textbooks which must be covered during the course of three or two years.

This thought is what motivated us to come up with a student friendly book which can be read and revised before you give your examinations. This is not aimed at just postgraduates who are giving examinations. Even a candidate who is getting introduced to the subject can read it as it covers more than 200 common topics, what is expected from a postgraduate student during ward rounds and preparatory tests. This book also contains a compilation of theory questions asked in MS and DNB examinations over the past 15 years delicately arranged in a topic-wise manner. This will help all examination going students cover their topics leaving no stone unturned and boost their confidence during theory examinations.

It comes handy for one to refer to this book, be a postgraduate or a consultant during busy duty hours in the casualty or outpatient department (OPD). We have referred standard textbooks to compile the exhaustive list of classifications of upper limb and lower limb trauma, classifications of pediatric trauma, congenital and regional conditions of upper limb and lower limb, diagnostic criteria for various conditions, orthopedic formulas, and radiological lines.

Orthopedic Navigator: An Orthopedic Guide for Postgraduates has got simple, easy to reproduce diagrams which are drawn by the authors. We suggest every postgraduate must carry this from the beginning of your course so that after reading standard textbooks revision can be quickly done without wasting time or searching for answers on the internet.

We hope our effort helps you achieve great success.

Jacob Ipe
Febin Ahamed PI
Jacob Eapen

Contents

1. Upper Limb Trauma 1
- Clavicle Fracture *1*
- Scapula Fractures *2*
- Proximal Humerus Fracture *3*
- Glenohumeral Dislocation *5*
- Intercondylar Humerus Fracture *6*
- Elbow Dislocation *7*
- Coronoid Fracture *7*
- Olecranon Fracture *8*
- Radial Head Classification *9*
- Monteggia Fracture *9*
- Galeazzi Fracture *11*
- Distal Radius Fracture *11*
- Scaphoid Fracture *12*
- Perilunate Dislocations and Fracture Dislocations *13*
- Triangular Fibrocartilage Injuries *14*
- Fingertip Injuries *15*

2. Lower Limb Trauma 17
- Pelvic Fractures *17*
- Acetabulum Fracture *18*
- Hip Dislocation *20*
- Head of Femur Fracture *21*
- Neck of Femur Fracture *22*
- Intertrochanteric Fractures *23*
- Subtrochanteric Femur Fractures *24*
- Femoral Shaft Fractures *25*
- Distal Femur Fracture *25*
- Patella Fracture Classification *26*
- Proximal Tibial Fractures *27*
- Floating Knee (Ipsilateral Fractures of Femur and Tibia) *28*
- Knee Dislocation (KD) *28*
- Tibiofibular Shaft Fractures *29*
- Foot and Ankle Fractures *30*
- Tibial Pilon Fracture *33*
- Talar Neck Fractures *34*
- Talar Body Fracture *34*

- Calcaneus Fracture *35*
- Lisfranc Fracture *35*
- Chopart Fracture *36*
- Navicular Fracture *36*
- 5th Metatarsal Fracture *37*

3. Pediatric Trauma 38
- Salter–Harris Physeal Injury *38*
- Proximal Humerus Fracture *39*
- Supracondylar Elbow Fracture *40*
- Lateral Condyle Humerus Physeal Fractures *41*
- Medial Condyle Humerus Physeal Fractures *41*
- Radial Head and Neck Fractures *42*
- Pediatric Pelvic Fracture *43*
- Fractures of the Neck of Femur *43*
- Tibial Tubercle Fractures *44*

4. Spine Trauma 45
- Spinal Cord Injury *45*
- American Spinal Injury Association (ASIA) Impairment Scale *45*
- Occipital Condyle Fracture *45*
- Atlanto-occipital Dislocation *46*
- Atlas Fracture (Jefferson's Fracture) *46*
- Atlantoaxial Rotatory Subluxation and Dislocation *47*
- Fractures of the Odontoid Process (DENS) *47*
- Traumatic Spondylolisthesis of C-2 (Hangman's Fracture) *48*
- Thoracolumbar Fractures *49*
- Sacral Fractures *50*

5. Upper Limb Regional Conditions 51
- Frozen Shoulder *51*
- Impingement Syndrome *51*
- Calcific Tendinitis *51*
- Superior Labrum Anterior and Posterior (SLAP) Tear *52*
- Dupuytren's Contracture *53*
- Trigger Finger *53*
- Brachial Plexus Injury *53*
- Rotator Cuff Tears *54*
- Elbow Instability *55*
- Scaphoid Lunate Advanced Collapse (SLAC) *56*
- Perilunate Dislocation *57*
- Kienbock's Disease *57*
- Reflex Sympathetic Dystrophy (RSD) *58*

6. Lower Limb Regional Conditions 59
- Perthes Disease *59*
- Slipped Capital Femoral Epiphysis *63*
- Developmental Dysplasia of Hip *63*
- Avascular Necrosis *65*
- Femoroacetabular Impingement *67*
- Osteoarthritis *67*
- Chondromalacia Patella *68*
- Bipartite Patella *69*
- Accessory Navicular *69*
- Hallux Valgus *70*
- Osteochondritis Dissecans of Talus *70*
- Diabetic Foot *71*
- Charcot's Arthropathy *71*
- Tendoachilles Disorders *72*
- Tibialis Posterior Insufficiency *72*

7. Spinal Disorders 73
- Lumbar Canal Stenosis *73*
- Spondylolisthesis *73*
- Kyphosis *75*
- Intervertebral Disk Prolapse *75*
- Spinal Tuberculosis *76*

8. Congenital Anomalies 78
- Winging of Scapula *78*
- Sprengel's Shoulder *78*
- Torticollis *79*
- Congenital Radioulnar Synostosis *79*
- Congenital Hand Anomalies *80*
- Radial Club Hand *81*
- Thumb Anomaly Types *81*
- Hypoplasia of Thumb *82*
- Syndactyly *82*
- Apert Syndrome *82*
- Ring Constriction Syndrome *83*
- Ulnar Club Hand *83*
- Madelung Deformity *83*
- Proximal Femoral Focal Deficiency *84*
- Blount's Disease/Congenital Tibia Vara *84*
- Congenital Pseudarthrosis of Tibia *85*
- Congenital Talipes Equinovarus *87*

- Congenital Vertical Talus *88*
- Tibia Hemimelia *88*
- Fibular Hemimelia *89*

9. Miscellaneous Conditions 90

- Open Fracture *90*
- Gait *91*
- Mangled Extremity Severity Score (MESS) *91*
- Injury Severity Score *92*
- Ganga Hospital Scoring System *92*
- Glasgow Coma Scale (GCS) *93*
- Nonunion *94*
- Femur Neck Nonunion *96*
- Osteomyelitis *96*
- Septic Arthritis Sequelae *97*
- Pin Tract Site Infection *99*
- Malignant Tumor *99*
- Hereditary Multiple Exostoses *100*
- Giant Cell Tumor *100*
- Pattern of Bone Destruction *101*
- Periprosthetic Fracture of Hip *101*
- Periprosthetic Fracture around Knee *102*
- Periprosthetic Infection *103*
- Limb Length Discrepancy *103*
- Functional Classification of Rheumatoid Arthritis *103*
- Heterotopic Ossification of Elbow *103*
- Osteogenesis Imperfecta (OI) *104*
- Hemophilia *104*

10. Diagnostic Criteria 105

- Kanavel's Sign *105*
- Kocher Criteria *105*
- Morrey and Peterson's Criteria *105*
- Peltola and Vahvanen's Criteria *105*
- Rheumatoid Arthritis *106*
- Ankylosing Spondylitis *106*
- Mirels' Criteria *107*
- Spine at Risk *107*
- Juvenile Rheumatoid Arthritis (JRA) *107*
- Diffuse Idiopathic Skeletal Hyperostosis *108*
- Neurofibromatosis *108*
- Spine Instability *108*
- Multiple Myeloma *109*

- Fat Embolism *109*
- Hyperlaxity *110*
- Adult Respiratory Distress Syndrome *110*

11. Formulas in Orthopedics 111
- Biomechanics of Hip *111*
- Baumgartner Index (Tip-Apex Distance) *111*
- Osteotomy Wedge *111*
- Change in Length after Osteotomy *112*
- Menelaus Method (Limb Length Discrepancy) *112*
- Calculation of Nail Size (Pediatric) *112*
- Ilizarov Lengthening *112*
- Tibial Tuberosity Index *113*
- Radial Bow Calculation *113*
- Insall–Salvati Index *113*
- Tourniquet Pressure *113*
- Flexibility Index (Scoliosis) *114*
- Tuberculosis Spine (Calculation of Final Deformity) *114*

12. Radiological Lines 115
- Shoulder *115*
- Elbow *116*
- Wrist *119*
- Hip *123*
- Knee *128*
- Ankle *132*
- Foot *135*
- Spine *136*

13. DNB Practical Examination 148

Question Bank 155
- Basic Sciences and General Orthopedics *155*
- Arthrodesis *157*
- Arthroplasty *157*
- Amputation *159*
- Infections *159*
- Tumor *161*
- Congenital/Developmental Anomalies *162*
- Pediatric Orthopedics *163*
- Neuromuscular Disorders *164*

- Fracture and Dislocation *165*
- Spine *169*
- Sports Medicine *171*
- Nerve Injuries *172*
- Microsurgery *173*
- Hand and Wrist *173*
- Foot and Ankle *174*
- Hip and Pelvis *175*
- Arthropathy and Inflammatory Disorders *175*
- Investigations and Clinical Tests *176*
- Orthotics and Prosthesis *176*
- Implants and Surgical Techniques *177*
- Physiotherapy *179*
- Metabolic Disorders *179*
- PSM *180*
- Miscellaneous *180*

Index 183

CHAPTER 1

Upper Limb Trauma

CLAVICLE FRACTURE

Allman Classification

- *Group 1:* Fracture of the middle third

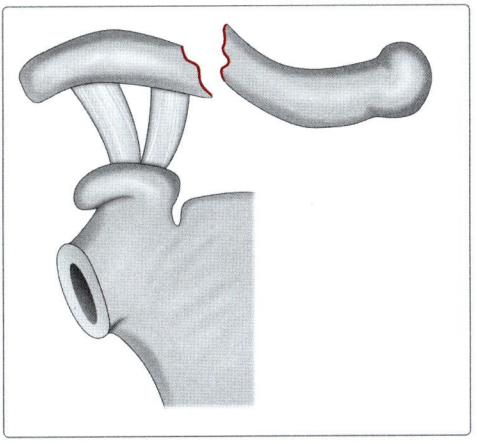

- *Group 2:* Fracture of distal segment
  - *Type 1:* Displaced secondary to a fracture medial to the coracoclavicular (CC) ligaments
  - *Type 2:* Conoid and trapezoid attached to the proximal segment
  - *Type 3:* Conoid torn and trapezoid attached

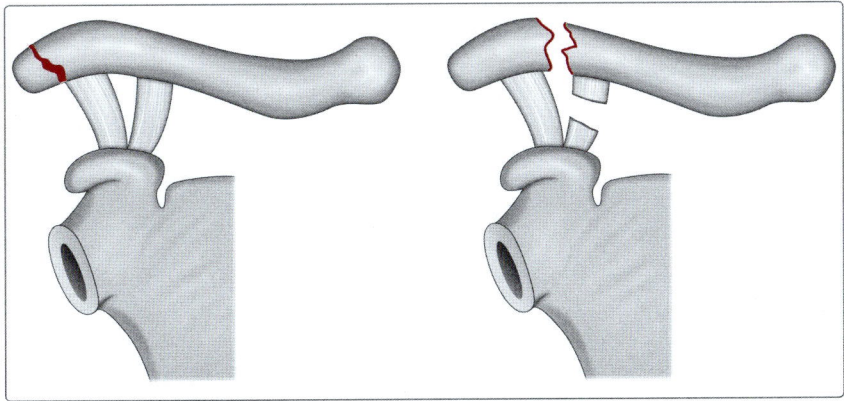

- *Group 3:* Fracture of proximal third
  - *Type 1:* Minimal displacement
  - *Type 2:* Displaced
  - *Type 3:* Intra-articular
  - *Type 4:* Epiphyseal separation
  - *Type 5:* Comminuted

SCAPULA FRACTURES

Ideberg Classification (Intra-articular Glenoid Fracture)

- *Type 1:* Avulsion fracture of the anterior margin
- *Type 2a:* Transverse fracture through the glenoid fossa exiting inferiorly
- *Type 2b:* Oblique fracture through the glenoid fossa inferiorly
- *Type 3:* Oblique fracture through the glenoid fracture through the glenoid exiting superiorly; often associated with an acromioclavicular (AC) joint injury
- *Type 4:* Transverse fracture exiting through the medial border of the scapula
- *Type 5:* Combination of a type 2 and type 4 pattern

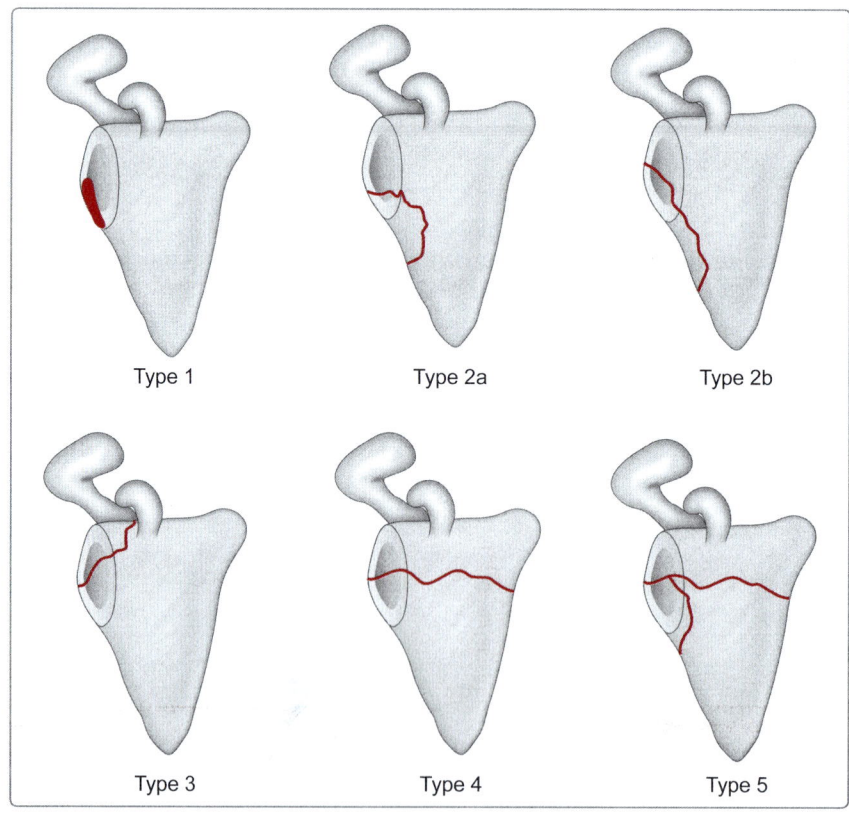

Upper Limb Trauma

Acromioclavicular Joint Injuries
Rockwood Classification
- *Type 1:* Sprain of the AC ligament
- *Type 2:* AC ligament tear and CC ligaments sprained
- *Type 3:* AC and CC ligaments torn
- *Type 4:* Type 3 with distal clavicle displaced posteriorly into or through the trapezius
- *Type 5:* Type 3 with the distal clavicle grossly displaced superiorly
- *Type 6:* AC dislocated with the clavicle displaced inferior to the acromion or coracoid

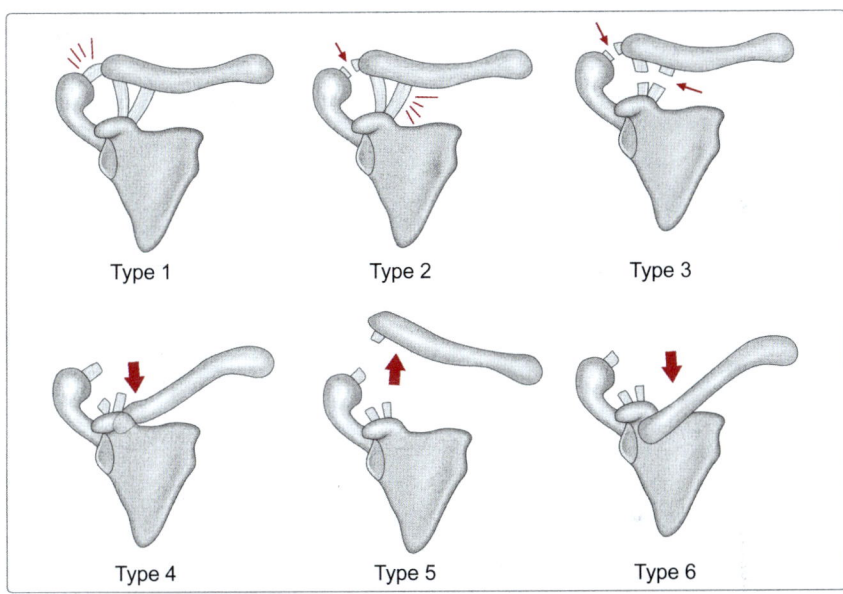

PROXIMAL HUMERUS FRACTURE

Neer Classification
- Minimally displaced or undisplaced fracture

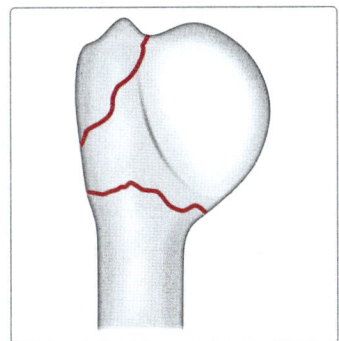

- *2-part fracture:* It may be greater tuberosity fracture, lesser tuberosity fracture, surgical neck fracture or anatomical neck fracture.

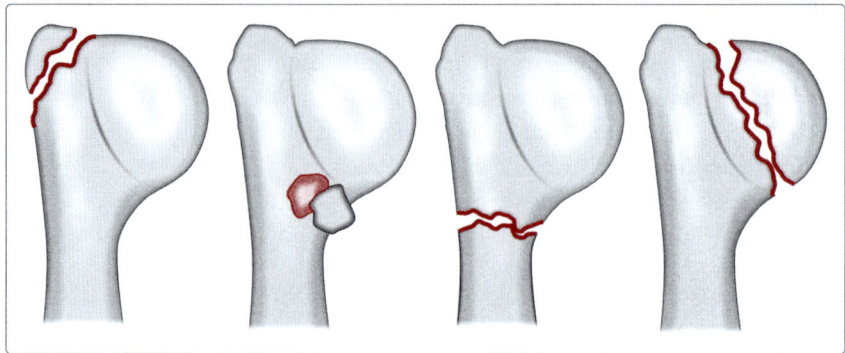

- *3-part fracture:* Usually the fragments are—greater tuberosity and surgical neck; lesser tuberosity and surgical neck

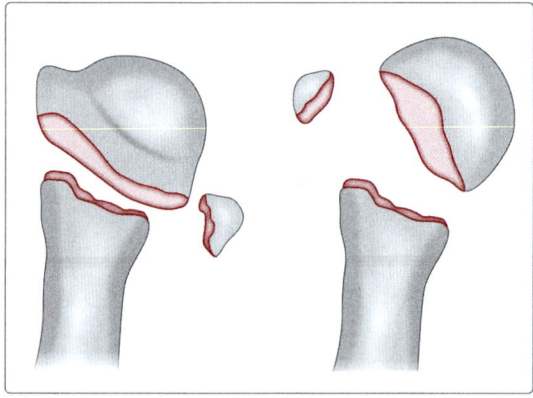

- *4-part fracture:* The four parts are greater and lesser tuberosities, shaft and humeral head.

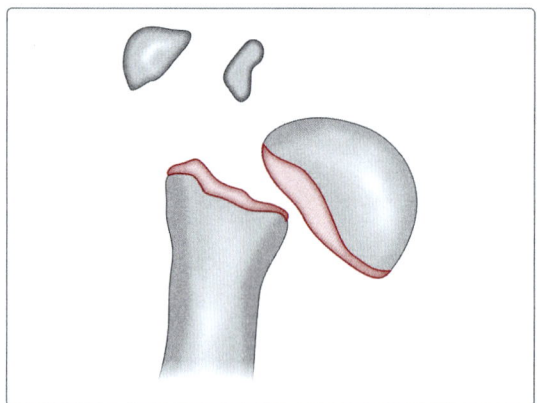

GLENOHUMERAL DISLOCATION

Anatomical Classification

- Anterior dislocation
- Inferior dislocation (Luxatio erecta)
- Posterior dislocation
- Superior dislocation

Anterior Dislocation

- Subclavicular
- Subcoracoid
- Intrathoracic

Posterior Dislocation

- Subacromial
- Subglenoid
- Subspinous

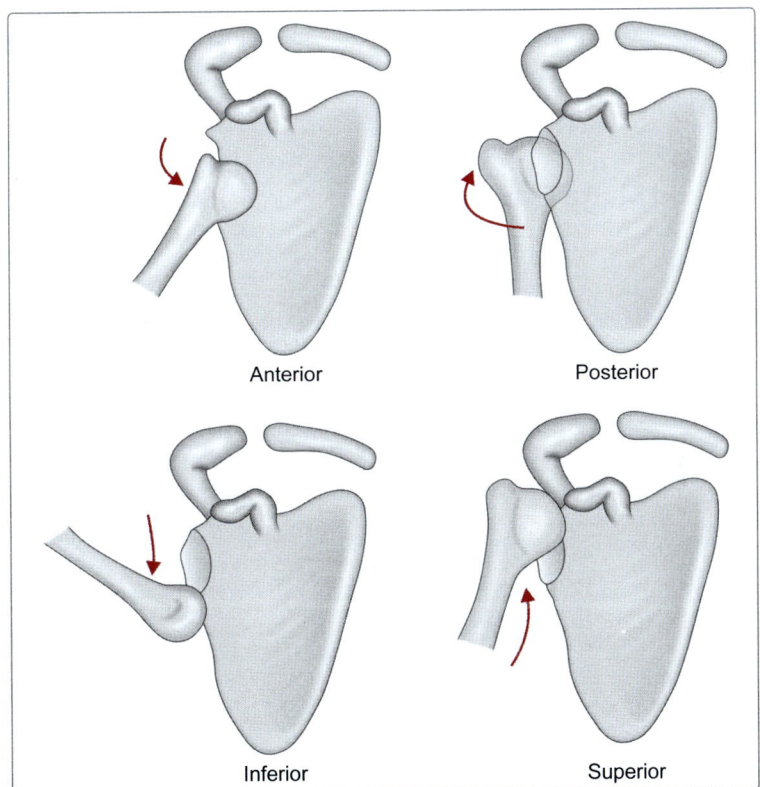

Recurrent Shoulder Dislocation

Matsen's Classification

This classification is for recurrent shoulder dislocation.
- *TUBS:* Traumatic unilateral, with a Bankart's lesion, requires surgery
- *AMBRII:* Atraumatic, multidirectional and bilateral, responds to rehabilitation occasionally requires an inferior capsular shift and internal closure.

INTERCONDYLAR HUMERUS FRACTURE

Riseborough and Radin Classification

- *Type 1:* Nondisplaced
- *Type 2:* Slight displacement with no rotation between the condylar fragment
- *Type 3:* Displacement with rotation
- *Type 4:* Severe comminution of the articular surface

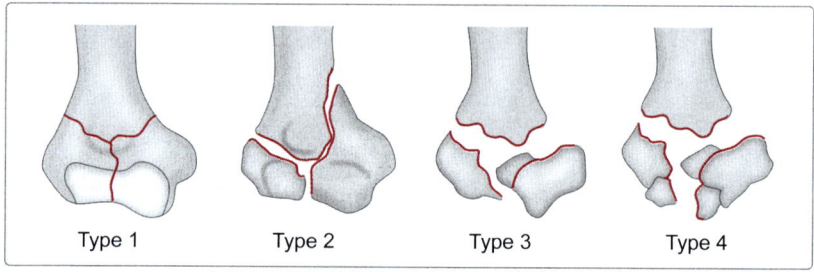

Mehne and Matta Classification

- High T
- Y-type
- Medial
- Low T
- H-type
- Lateral

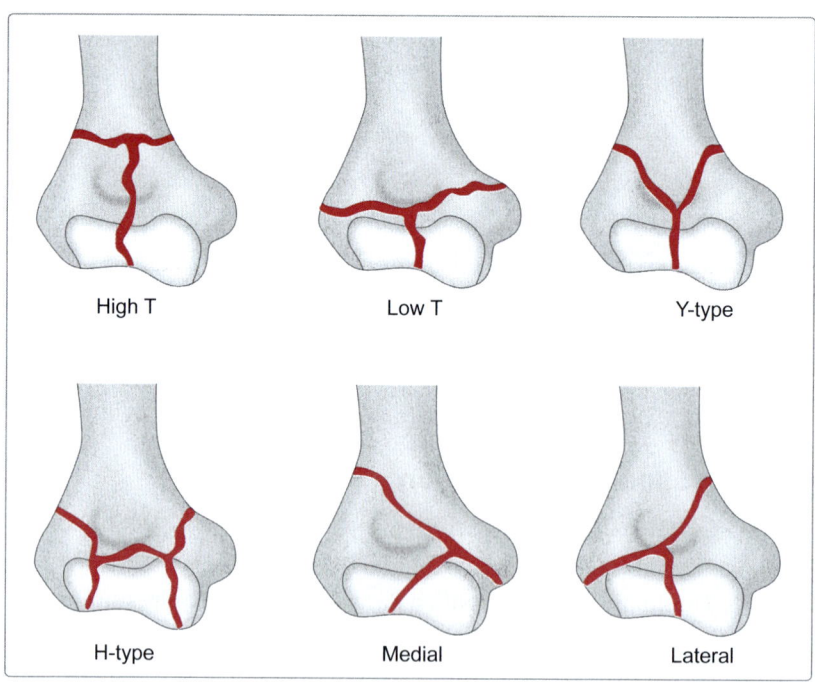

ELBOW DISLOCATION

Anatomical Classification

- Posterior
  - *Posterolateral:* >90% dislocations
  - Posteromedial
- Anterior
- Medial
- Lateral
- Divergent (rare)

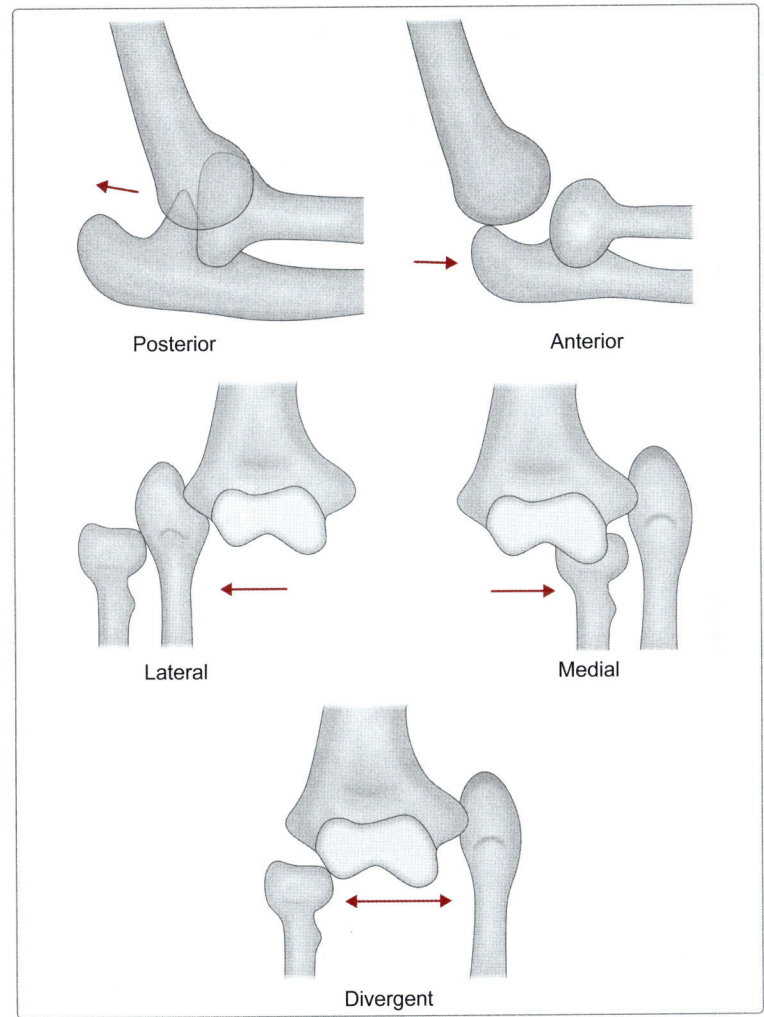

CORONOID FRACTURE

Regan and Morrey Classification

- *Type I:* Avulsion of the tip of the coronoid process

- *Type II:* Involving <50% of the process
- *Type III:* Involving >50% of the process, there may be an associated valgus instability, since medial collateral ligament inserts onto the fracture fragment.

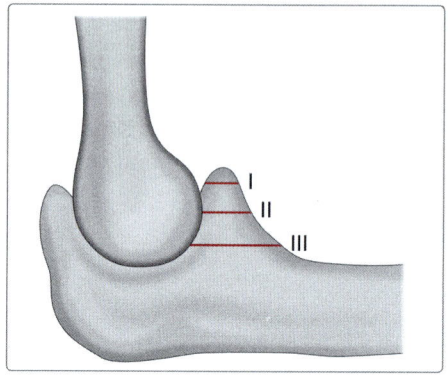

OLECRANON FRACTURE

Mayo Classification

- *Types 1A and 1B:* Undisplaced (>2 mm) fractures with no comminution (type 1A) or with comminution (type 1B)
- *Type 2A:* Stable fracture with 3 mm displacement, no comminution
- *Type 2B:* Stable fractures with 3 mm displacement; comminution is present.
- *Type 3:* Unstable, displaced fracture–dislocations; no comminution is present.

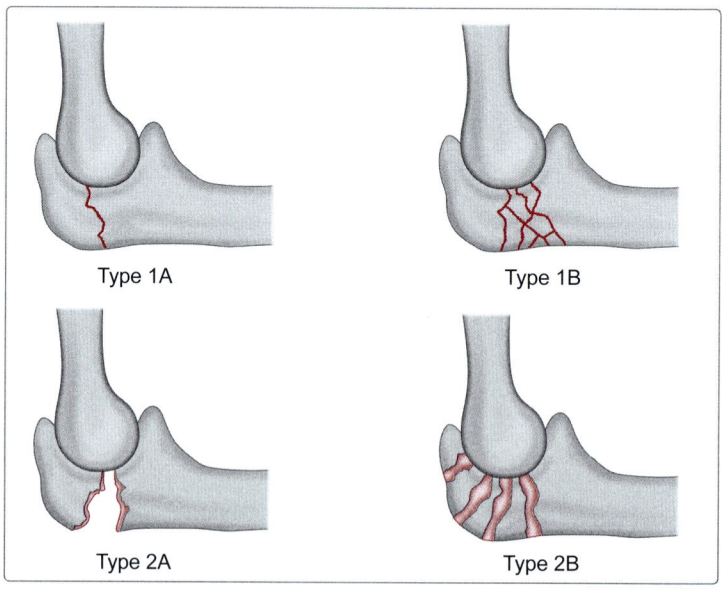

Upper Limb Trauma

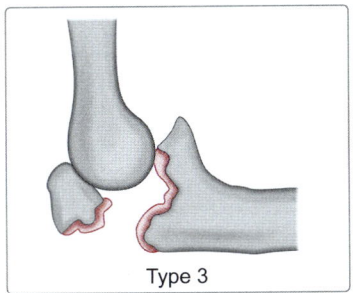
Type 3

RADIAL HEAD CLASSIFICATION

Mason Classification

- *Type 1:* Nondisplaced fractures
- *Type 2:* Marginal fractures with displacement
- *Type 3:* Comminuted fractures involving the entire head
- *Type 4:* Associated with dislocation of the elbow

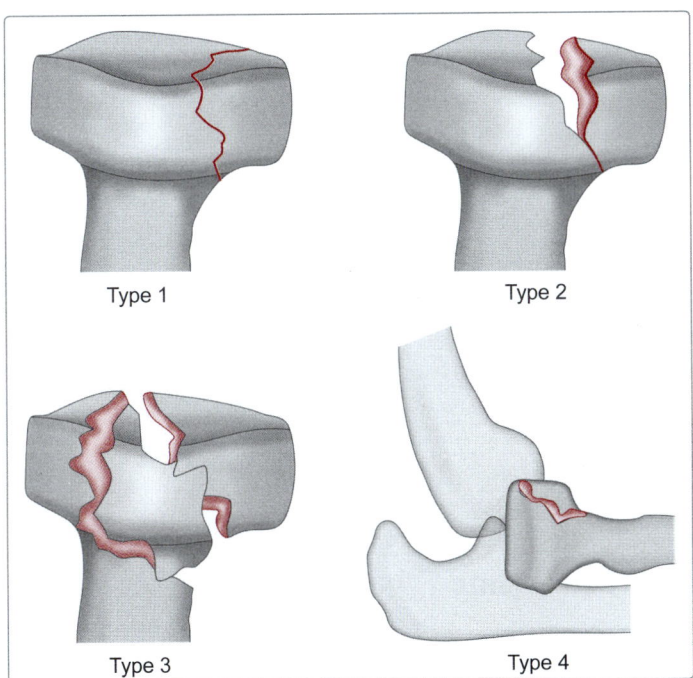

MONTEGGIA FRACTURE

Bado Classification

- *Type 1:* Anterior dislocation of the radial head with fracture of the ulnar diaphysis at any level with anterior angulation

- *Type 2:* Posterior/posterolateral dislocation of the radial head with fracture of the ulnar diaphysis with posterior angulation
- *Type 3:* Lateral/anterolateral dislocation of the radial head with fracture of the ulnar metaphysis
- *Type 4:* Anterior dislocation of the radial head with fractures of the both the radius and ulna within proximal third at the same level

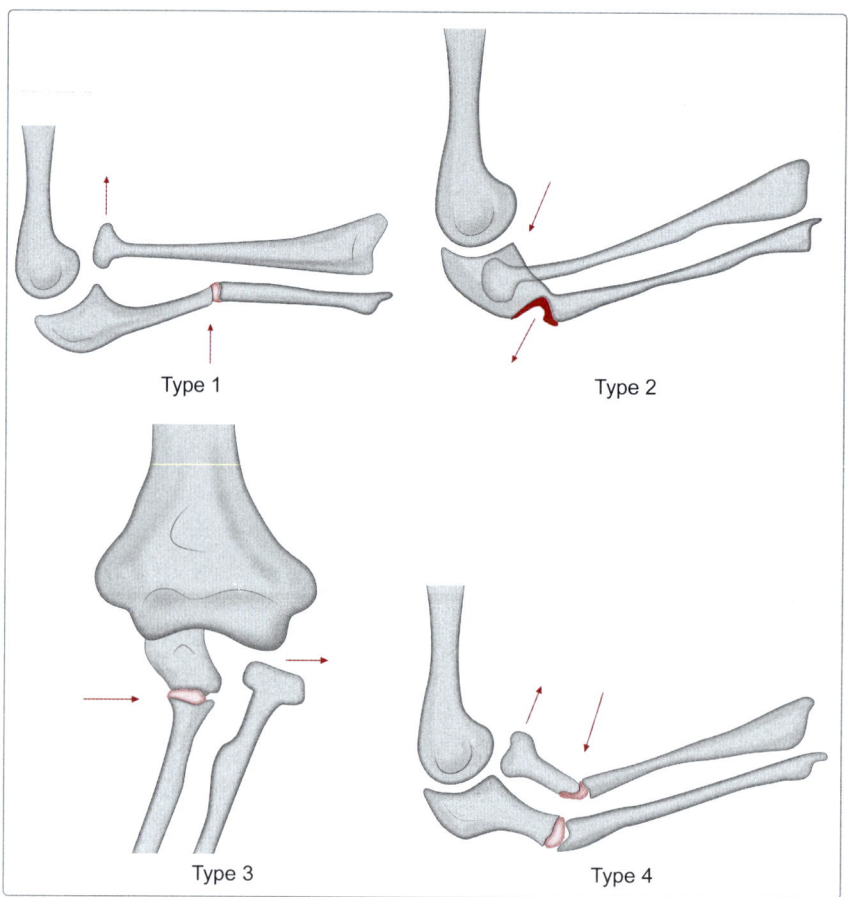

Monteggia Equivalents

- *Type I equivalents:*
  - Isolated dislocation of radial head
  - Radial neck fracture (isolated)
  - Radial neck fracture in combination with a fracture of the ulnar diaphysis
  - Radial and ulnar fractures with the radial fracture above the junction of the middle and proximal thirds
  - Fracture of ulnar diaphysis with anterior dislocation of radial head and an olecranon fracture.

- *Type II equivalents:* Fractures of the proximal radial epiphysis or radial neck.
- *Type III and Type IV equivalents:* Fractures of the distal humerus in association with proximal forearm fractures.

Letts' Classification of Pediatric Monteggia Fractures
- *Type A* (Plastic deformation of ulna)
- *Type B* (Greenstick fracture of ulna)
- *Type C* (Ulna complete fracture) is analogous to Bado type-I
- *Type D* is analogous to Bado type-II
- *Type E* is analogous to Bado type-III

GALEAZZI FRACTURE

Maculé–Beneyto Classification
Based on the location of radius fracture from the styloid.
- *Type 1:* 60% of the fractures were located within 10 cm from the styloid.
- *Type 2:* 30% of the fractures were located 10–15 cm from the styloid.
- *Type 3:* 10% of the fractures were >15 cm from the styloid.

DISTAL RADIUS FRACTURE

Fernandez Classification
- *Type 1 (Bending injury):* Colles' fracture and Smith fracture
- *Type 2 (Shear injury):* Volar Barton and Dorsal Barton
- *Type 3 (Impaction injury):* Complex articular fractures and radial pilon fracture
- *Type 4 (Avulsion):* Radiocarpal fracture dislocations
- *Type 5 (High velocity):* High-velocity injuries

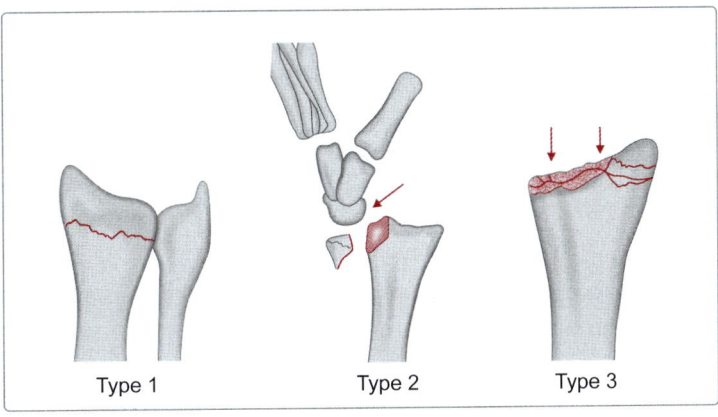

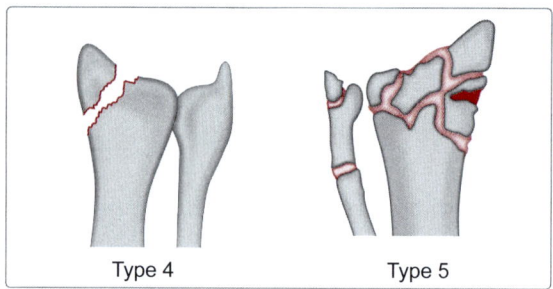

Type 4   Type 5

Frykman Classification

FRYKMAN CLASSIFICATION		
	Ulnar styloid fracture	
Radius fracture	Absent	Present
Extra-articular	1a	2a
Intra-articular involving radiocarpal joint	1b	2b
Intra-articular involving distal radioulnar joint (DRUJ)	1c	2c
Intra-articular involving radiocarpal and DRUJ	1d	2d

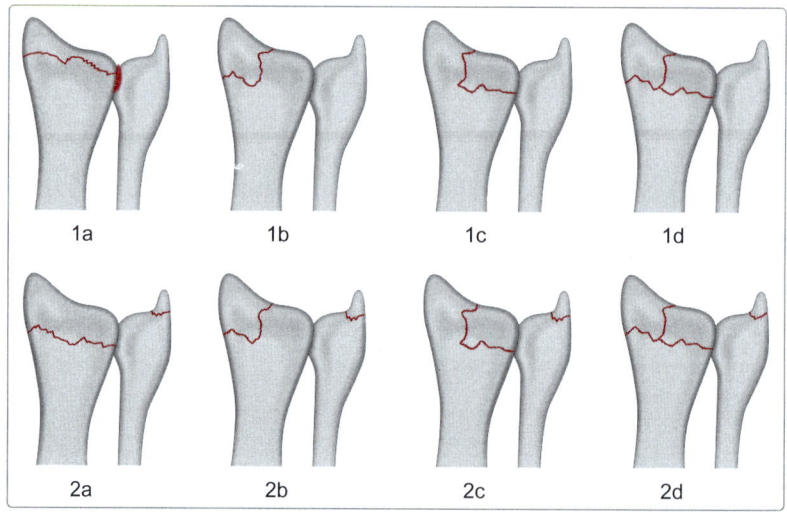

SCAPHOID FRACTURE

Herbert Classification

- Type A: Fractures include:
  - A1: Fractures of the tubercle
  - A2: Incomplete fractures through the waist, which are inherently stable

- *Type B:* Fractures are acute and unstable; they include:
  - *B1:* Distal oblique fractures
  - *B2:* Complete fractures through the waist
  - *B3:* Proximal pole fractures
  - *B4:* Transscaphoid perilunate fracture—dislocations of the carpus
- *Type C:* Delayed unions
- *Type D:* Established nonunion

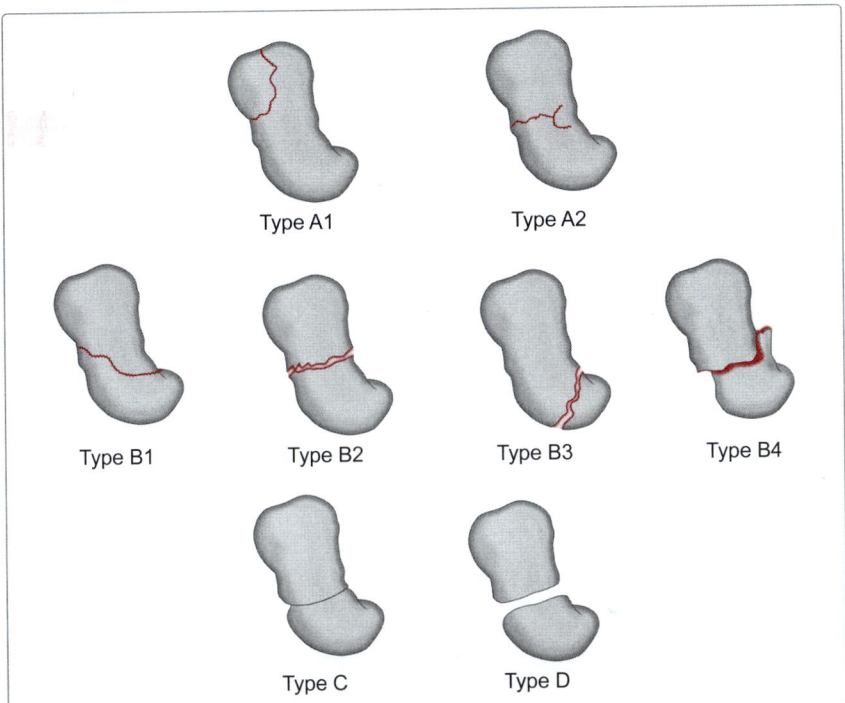

PERILUNATE DISLOCATIONS AND FRACTURE DISLOCATIONS

- *Greater arc:* A greater arc injury passes through the scaphoid, capitate and triquetrum and often results in trans-scaphoid transcapitate perilunate fracture dislocations.
- *Lesser arc:* A lesser arc injury follows a curved path through the radial styloid, midcarpal joint and lunotriquetral space and results in perilunate and lunate dislocations.

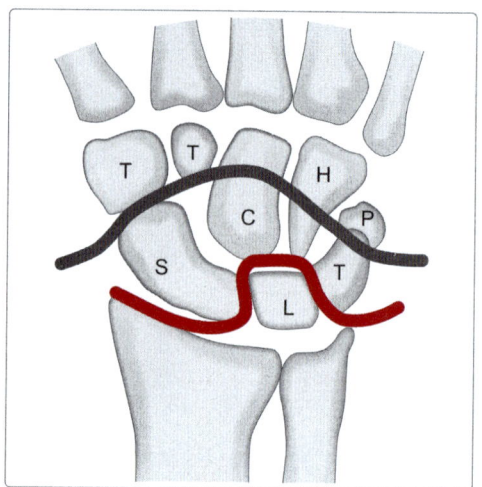

Note: Gilula's lines are three arcs drawn on an AP radiograph of the wrist used to assess the alignment of the carpal bones. There should be no step-off in the contour of the lines when drawn on a normal wrist.
- *First arc* running along the proximal convexity of the scaphoid, lunate and triquetrum.
- *Second arc* running along the distal concavities of the scaphoid, lunate and triquetrum.
- *Third arc* running along the proximal curvatures of the capitate and hamate.

TRIANGULAR FIBROCARTILAGE INJURIES

Class	Characteristics
	CLASSIFICATION OF TRAUMATIC TRIANGULAR FIBROCARTILAGE COMPLEX (TFCC) INJURIES
1A	Central perforation or tear
1B	Ulnar avulsion with or without ulnar styloid fracture
1C	Distal avulsion (origins of UL and UT ligaments)
1D	Radial avulsion (involving the dorsal and/or volar radioulnar ligaments)

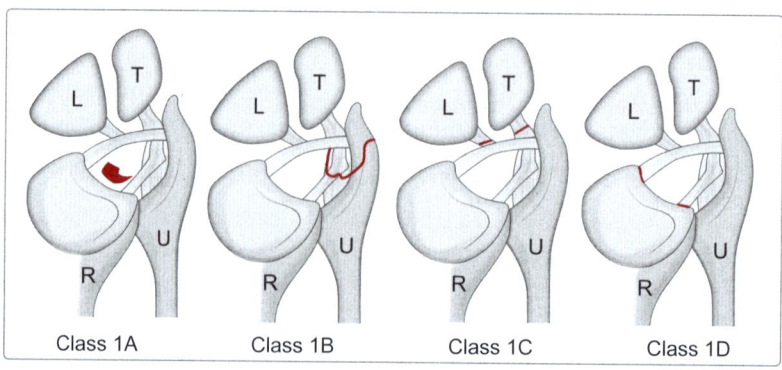

Class 1A   Class 1B   Class 1C   Class 1D

CLASSIFICATION OF DEGENERATIVE TRIANGULAR FIBROCARTILAGE COMPLEX (TFCC) TEARS

Class	Characteristics
2A	TFCC wear
2B	2A + Lunate or ulnar chondromalacia
2C	TFCC perforation + lunate and/or ulnar chondromalacia
2D	2C + LT ligament disruption
2E	2D + Ulnocarpal and DRUJ arthritis

(DRUJ: distal radioulnar joint)

FINGERTIP INJURIES

Allen Classification

- *Type I:* Injuries involve only the pulp
- *Type II:* Injuries involve the pulp and nail bed
- *Type III:* Injuries include partial loss of the distal phalanx
- *Type IV:* Injuries are proximal to the lunula

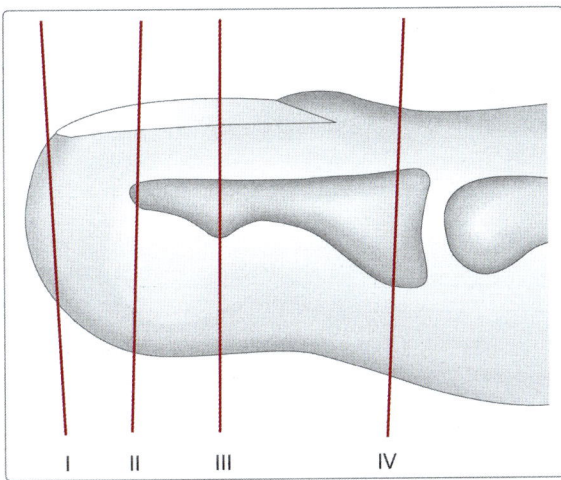

Mallet Finger

Doyle Classification

- *Type 1:* It is a tendinous rupture from the distal phalanx.
- *Type 2:* It is a tendinous laceration at or proximal to the DIP joint.
- *Type 3:* It is a deep abrasion with loss of extensor substance.
- *Type 4:* It includes a significant fracture of the distal phalanx.

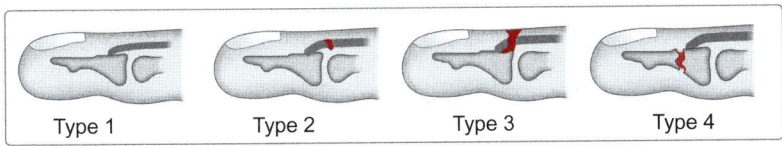

Jersey Finger

Leddy Classification

- *Type 1:* Tendon retracts into the palm with or without a bony fragment.
- *Type 2 (most common):* The tendon retracts to the proximal interphalangeal joint and the long vinculum remains intact. Type 1 and type 2 injuries may have a small bony avulsion.
- *Type 3:* Injuries involve a large bony fragment.

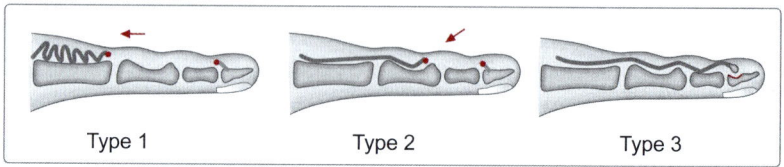

Fractures of Base of Thumb

- Extra-articular fractures
- *Intra-articular fractures (Rolando and Bennett fracture):* Rolando is comminuted intra-articular fracture, whereas, Bennett fracture is simple intra-articular fracture.

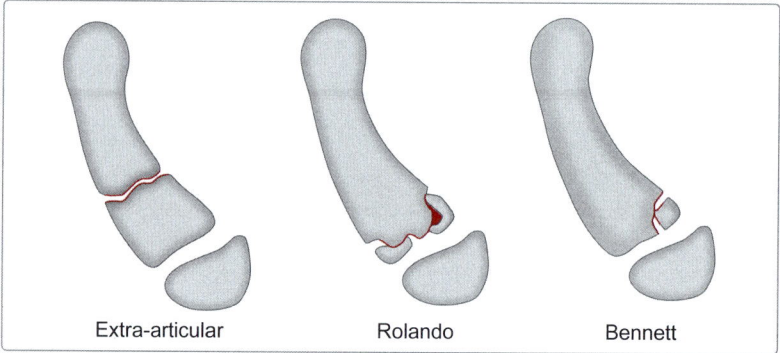

CHAPTER 2

Lower Limb Trauma

PELVIC FRACTURES

Tile Classification

- *Type A:* Stable (posterior arch intact)
  - *A1:* Fracture not involving the ring (avulsion of iliac wing fracture)
  - *A2:* Stable or minimally displaced fracture of the ring, e.g., isolated pubic ramus fracture
  - *A3:* Transverse sacral fracture (Denis zone III sacral fracture)

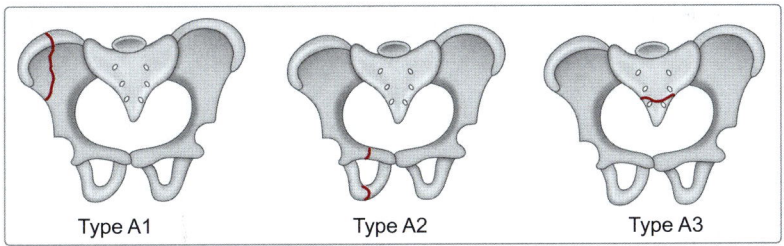

- *Type B:* Rotationally unstable, vertically stable (incomplete disruption of posterior arch)
  - *B1:* Open-book injury (external rotation), e.g., symphyseal diastasis
  - *B2:* Lateral compression injury (internal rotation), e.g., fracture of both pubic rami on the same side
    - *B2-1:* With anterior ring rotation/displacement through ipsilateral rami
    - *B2-2:* With anterior ring rotation/displacement through contralateral rami (bucket-handle injury)
  - *B3:* Bilateral

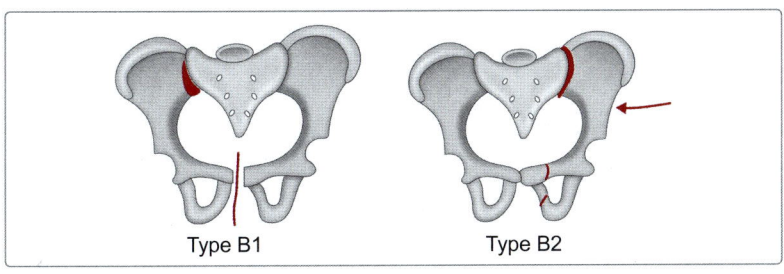

- *Type C:* Rotationally and vertically unstable
  - *C1:* Unilateral
    - *C1-1:* Iliac fracture
    - *C1-2:* Sacroiliac fracture-dislocation
    - *C1-3:* Sacral fracture
  - *C2:* Bilateral with one side type B and one side type C
  - *C3:* Bilateral with both sides

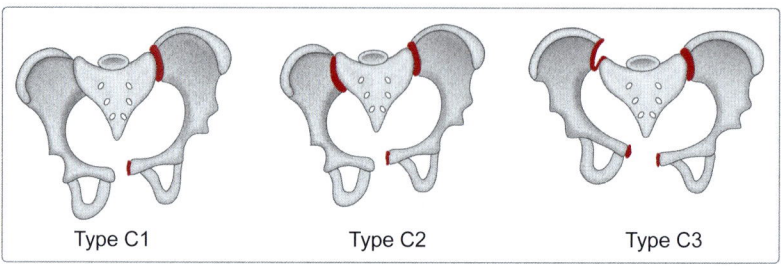

Young–Burgess Classification

- *Anterior-posterior compression (APC):*
  - *I*—symphysis widening <2.5 cm
  - *II*—symphysis widening >2.5 cm, anterior sacroiliac joint tear, posterior intact
  - *III*—disruption of both anterior and sacroiliac joints
- *Lateral compression (LC):*
  - *I*—ramus fracture + ipsilateral sacral alar compression fracture
  - *II*—rami fracture + ipsilateral posterior ilium fracture
  - *III*—ipsilateral LC (I/II) + contralateral APC
- *Vertical shear:* Posterior and superior directed force. [Associated with the highest risk of hypovolemic shock (63%); mortality rate up to 25%]
- Combined injury

ACETABULUM FRACTURE

Letournel and Judet Classification

Elementary (simple) fracture	Associated (combined)
Posterior wall	T-shaped
Posterior column	Anterior wall/column + posterior hemitransverse
Anterior wall	Transverse + posterior wall
Anterior column	Posterior column + posterior wall
Transverse	Both column

Lower Limb Trauma

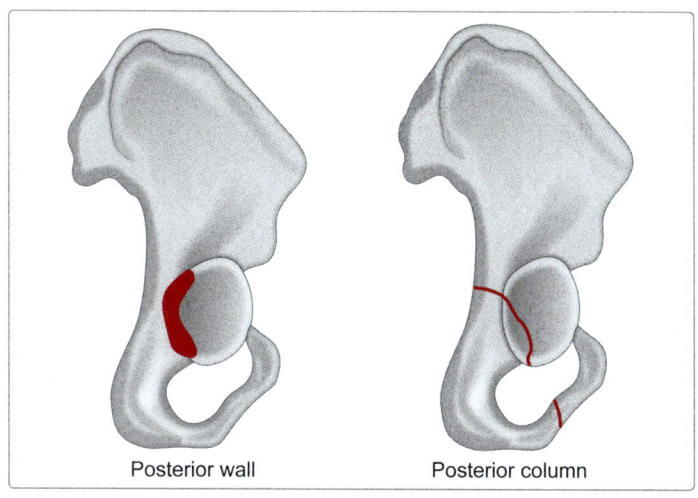

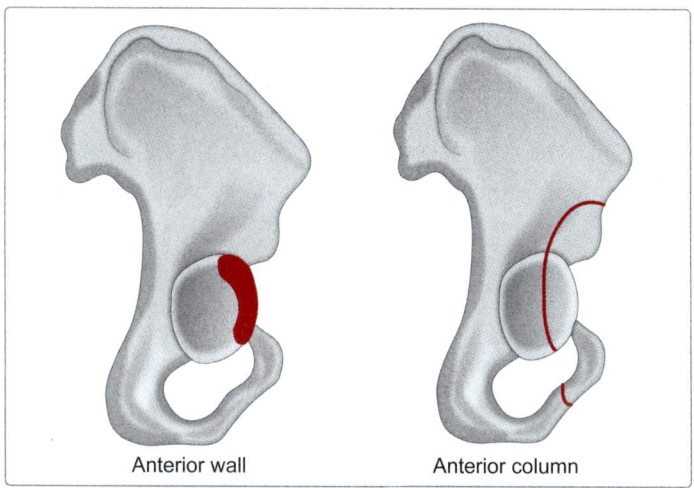

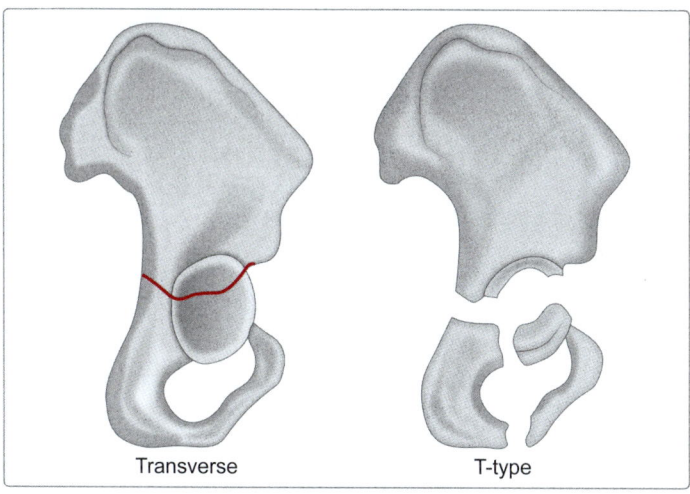

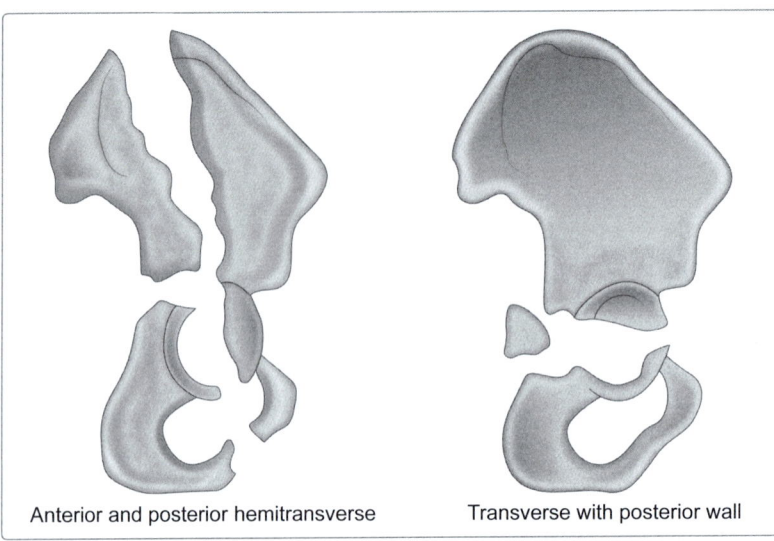

Anterior and posterior hemitransverse | Transverse with posterior wall

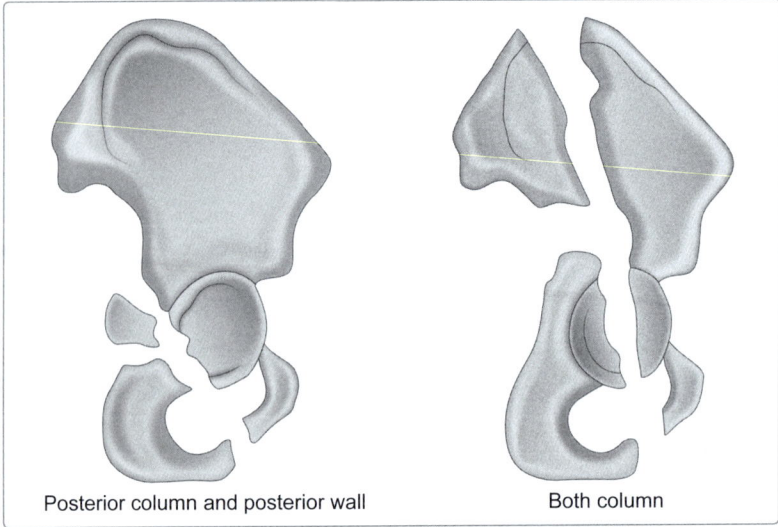

Posterior column and posterior wall | Both column

HIP DISLOCATION

Thompson and Epstein Classification

Posterior Dislocation
- *Type 1:* With or without a minor fracture
- *Type 2:* With large single fracture of posterior acetabular rim
- *Type 3:* With comminution of rim of acetabulum with or without major fracture
- *Type 4:* With fracture of the acetabular floor
- *Type 5:* With fracture of the femoral head

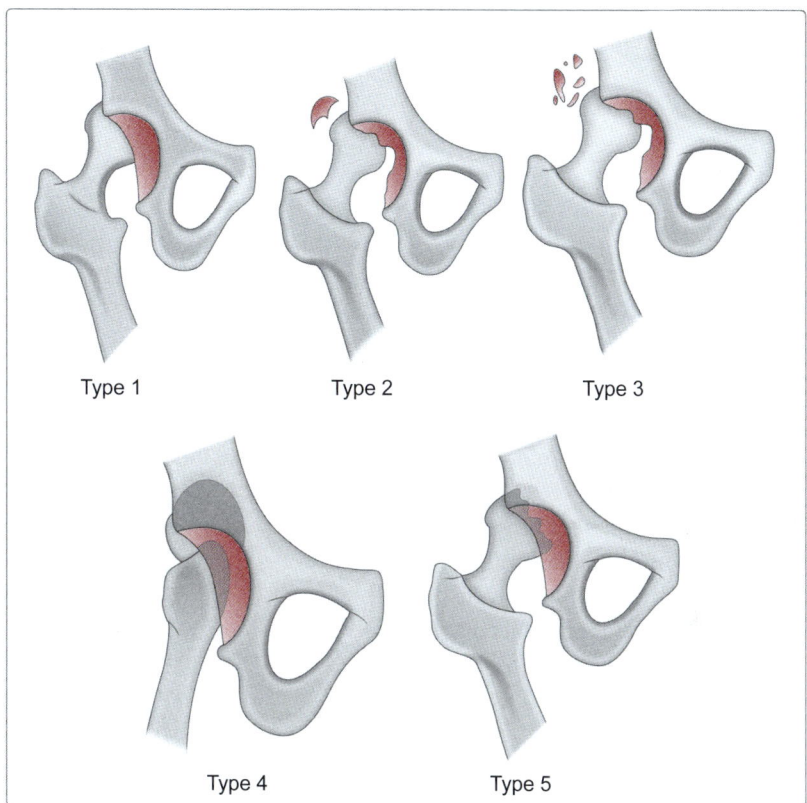

Epstein Classification

Anterior dislocation

- *Type I:* Superior dislocations (pubis and subspinous)
- *Type II:* Inferior dislocations (obturator and perineal)

Each type further subdivided into:
- *A:* Simple dislocation
- *B:* With femur head fracture
- *C:* With acetabulum fracture

HEAD OF FEMUR FRACTURE

Pipkin Classification

- *Type 1:* Fracture below the ligamentum teres
- *Type 2:* Fracture above the ligamentum involving weight-bearing area
- *Type 3:* Type 1 or 2 with fracture neck of femur
- *Type 4:* Type 1 or 2 with acetabular wall fracture (posterior wall)

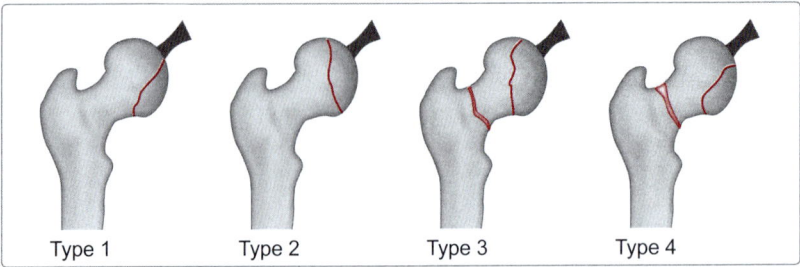

NECK OF FEMUR FRACTURE

Garden Classification

It is based on the completeness of the fracture and the displacement of trabecular alignment.
- *Type 1:* Incomplete, undisplaced
- *Type 2:* Complete, undisplaced
- *Type 3:* Complete, partially displaced
- *Type 4:* Complete, displaced completely

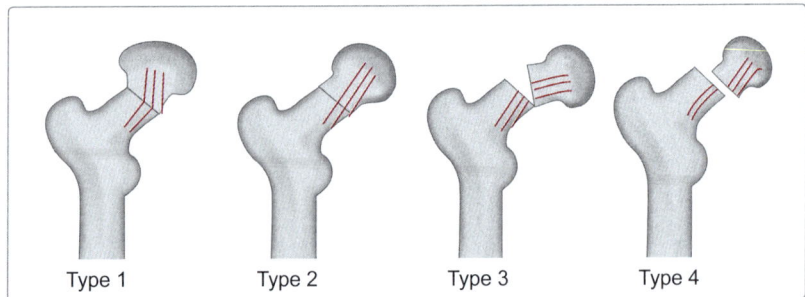

Pauwel's Classification

It is based on the angle the fracture line makes with the horizontal line through the pelvis.
- *Type 1:* <30%
- *Type 2:* 30–50%
- *Type 3:* >50%

Sandhu's Classification of Neglected Neck of Femur Fracture

- *Stage I:*
  - Fracture surfaces are still irregular (irregular or jagged).
  - The size of the proximal fragment is 2.5 cm or more.
  - The gap between the fragments is 1 cm or less.
  - Head of the femur is viable with no sign of AVN on X-ray or MRI.

- Stage II:
  - Fracture surfaces are smooth and sclerosed.
  - The size of the proximal fragment is 2.5 cm or more.
  - The gap between the fragments is more than 1 cm but <2.5 cm.
  - The head of the femur is viable.
- Stage III:
  - Fracture surfaces are smoothened out.
  - The size of the proximal fragment is <2.5 cm.
  - The gap between the fragments is more than 2.5 cm.
  - Signs of AVN seen.

INTERTROCHANTERIC FRACTURES

Boyd and Griffin Classification

- *Type I:* Linear intertrochanteric
- *Type II:* With comminution of trochanteric region
- *Type III:* With comminution associated with the subtrochanteric component
- *Type IV:* Reverse oblique fracture of the shaft with extension into the subtrochanteric region

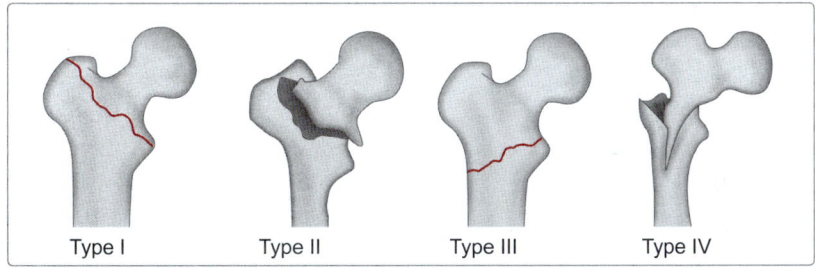

Evans Classification

- *Type I:* Fracture line extends upward and outward from the lesser trochanter *(stable)*.
  - *Type Ia:* Undisplaced two-fragment fracture
  - *Type Ib:* Displaced two-fragment fracture
  - *Type Ic:* Three-fragment fracture without posterolateral support, owing to displacement of greater trochanter fragment
  - *Type Id:* Three-fragment fracture without medial support, owing to displaced lesser trochanter or femoral arch fragment
  - *Type Ie:* Four-fragment fracture without posterolateral and medial support (combination of Type III and Type IV)
- *Type II:* Fracture line extends downward and outward from the lesser trochanter *(reverse obliquity/unstable)*. These fractures are unstable and have a tendency to drift medially.

SUBTROCHANTERIC FEMUR FRACTURES

Russell–Taylor Classification

It is based on extension of fracture line into piriformis fossa.
- *Type I:* Fractures do not extend into piriformis fossa.
  - *IA:* No communition of lesser trochanter
  - *IB:* Communition of lesser trochanter
- *Type II:* Fracture extends into piriformis fossa.
  - *IIA:* No communition of lesser trochanter
  - *IIB:* Communtion of lesser trochanter

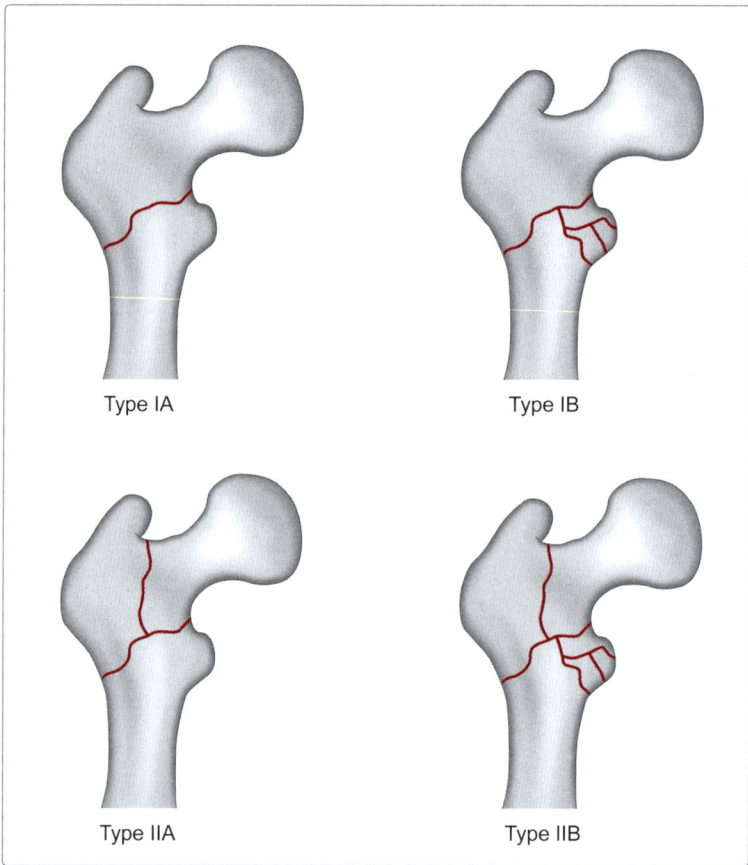

Fielding Classification

- *Type I:* At the level of the lesser trochanter (most common)
- *Type II:* Within the region 2.5 cm below the lesser trochanter
- *Type III:* Within the region 2.5–5 cm below the lesser trochanter (least common)

Seinsheimer Classification

SEINSHEIMER CLASSIFICATION		
Type I		Less than 2 mm displacement
Type II	A	2-part transverse fracture
	B	2-part spiral fracture with lesser trochanter attached to the proximal fragment
	C	2-part spiral fracture with lesser trochanter attached to the distal fragment
Type III	A	3-part spiral fracture with lesser trochanter as separate fragment
	B	3-part spiral fracture with butterfly fragment
Type IV		Comminuted fracture with four or more fragments
Type V		Fracture with proximal extension into the greater trochanter

FEMORAL SHAFT FRACTURES

Winquist and Hansen Classification

It is based on the cortical contact of proximal and distal fragment.
- *Type I:* Minimal communition, comminuted fragment <25% of width of femoral shaft
- *Type II:* Comminuted fragment involve 25–50%
- *Type III:* Comminuted fragment >50%, small contact between proximal and distal fragment
- *Type IV:* Communition involve the entire circumference, no cortical contact

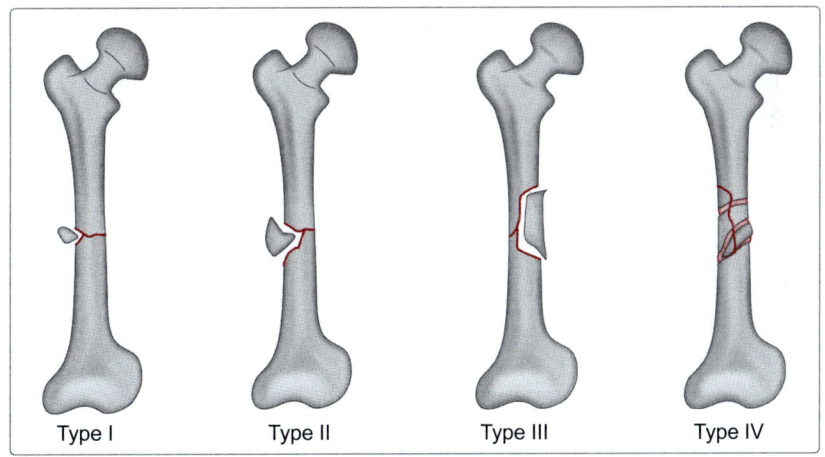

DISTAL FEMUR FRACTURE

Muller AO Classification

- *Type A:* Extra-articular fracture
  - *A1:* Simple

- *A2:* Metaphyseal wedge and/or fragmented wedge
- *A3:* Metaphyseal complex
- *Type B:* Partial articular fracture
  - *B1:* Lateral condyle, sagittal
  - *B2:* Medial condyle, sagittal
  - *B3:* Frontal/coronal plane fracture of condyles
- *Type C:* Complete articular fracture
  - *C1:* Articular simple, metaphyseal simple
  - *C2:* Articular simple, metaphyseal multifragmentary
  - *C3:* Articular multifragmentary

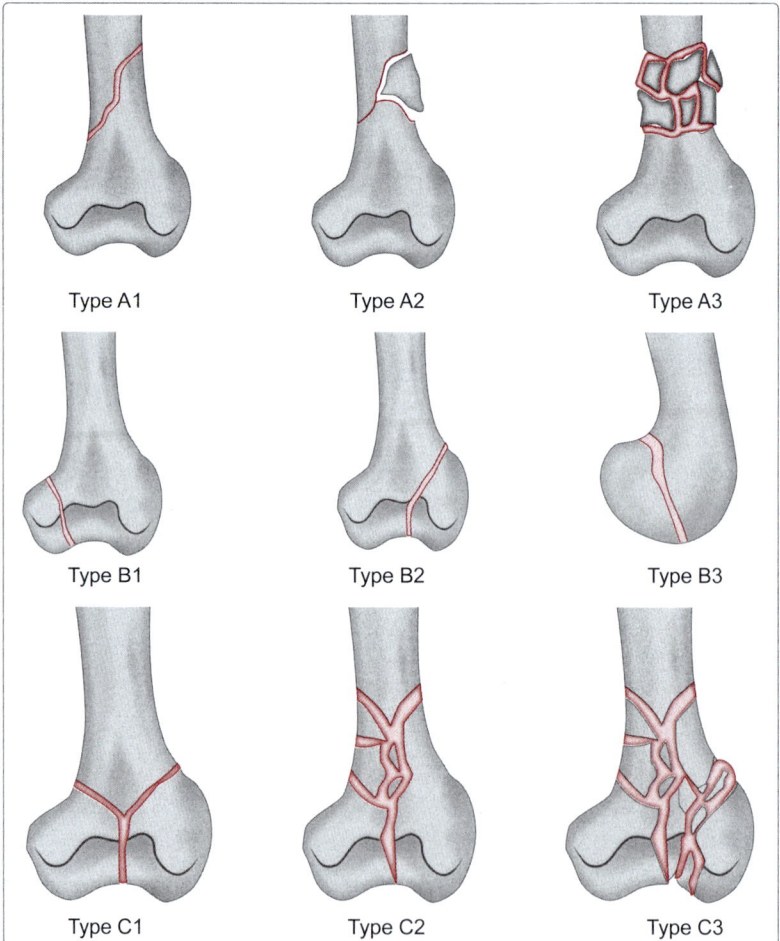

PATELLA FRACTURE CLASSIFICATION

It can be described based on fracture pattern:
- Nondisplaced
- Pole or sleeve (upper or lower)
- Transverse
- Vertical

- Marginal
- Comminuted (Stellate)
- Osteochondral

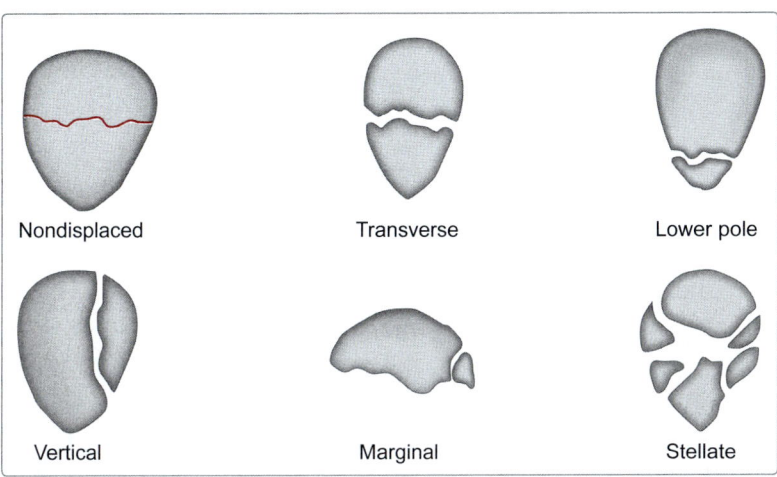

PROXIMAL TIBIAL FRACTURES

Schatzker Classification
- *Type I:* Lateral split fracture
- *Type II:* Split-depressed fracture of lateral plateau
- *Type III:* Pure depression fracture of lateral plateau
- *Type IV:* Medial plateau fracture
- *Type V:* Bicondylar fracture
- *Type VI:* Metaphyseal-diaphyseal disassociation

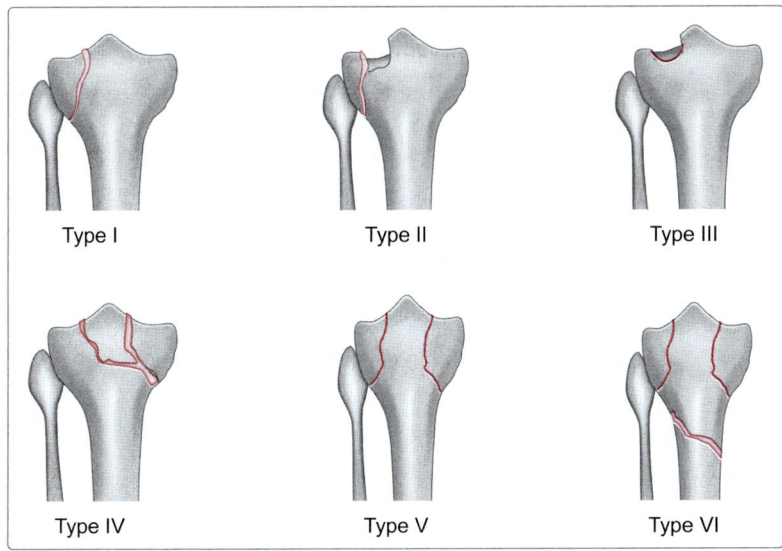

Hohl-Moore Classification

- *Type 1:* Coronal split fracture
- *Type 2:* Entire condylar fracture
- *Type 3:* Rim avulsion fracture of lateral plateau
- *Type 4:* Rim compression fracture
- *Type 5:* Four part fracture

FLOATING KNEE (IPSILATERAL FRACTURES OF FEMUR AND TIBIA)

Fraser Classification

- *Type I:* Extra-articular fractures
- *Type IIA:* Tibial plateau fracture and femoral shaft fracture
- *Type IIB:* Intra-articular distal femoral fracture and tibial shaft fracture
- *Type IIC:* Intra-articular fractures of both tibial plateau and distal femur

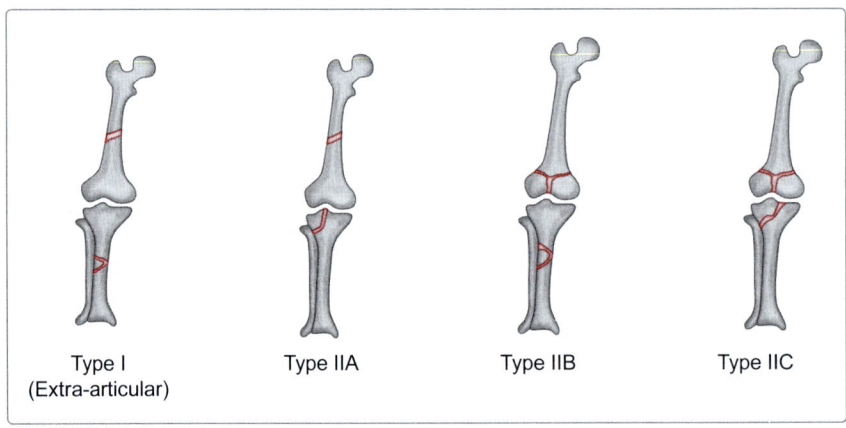

KNEE DISLOCATION (KD)

Schenck Classification

- *KD 1:* Single ligament injury (ACL or PCL)
- *KD 2:* Injury to ACL and PCL
- *KD 3:* Injury to ACL, PCL; with either MCL or LCL injury
  - *KD-3-M:* With MCL
  - *KD-3-L:* With LCL
- *KD 4:* With injury to ACL, PCL, MCL, LCL
- *KD 5:* Multiligamentous injury with periarticular fracture

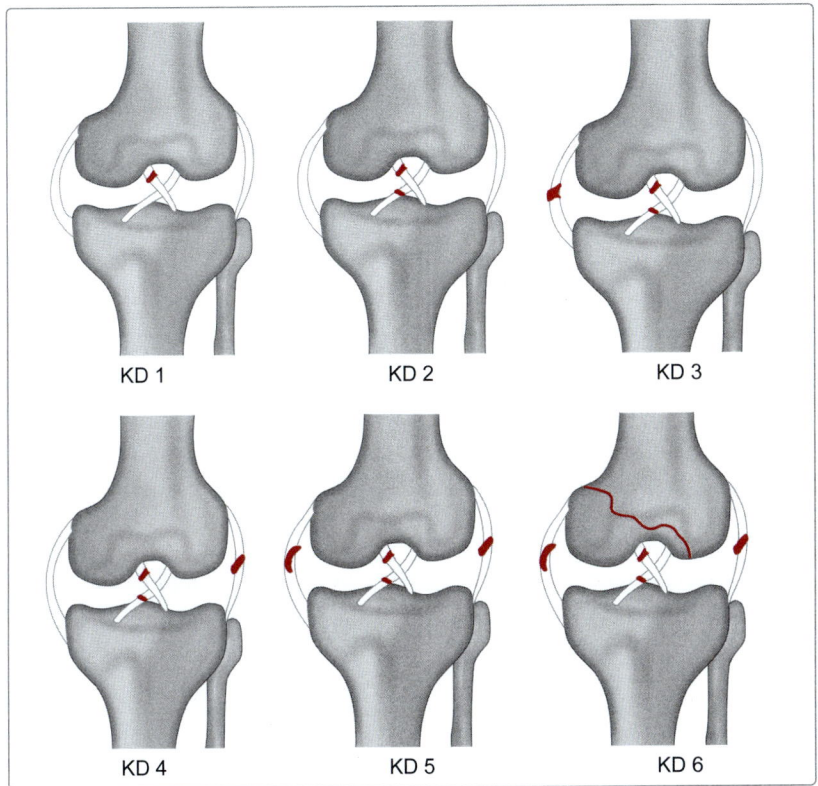

TIBIOFIBULAR SHAFT FRACTURES

AO Classification

A modification of *Johner and Wruh's* classification. It is still named as such by some authors.

Similar to AO classification of radioulnar, humeral, and femoral shaft fractures.
- *A:* Simple
- *B:* Wedge
- *C:* Complex

Modified Ellis Classification of Tibial Fractures

The system incorporates soft tissue injury grading by Gustilo-Anderson (open) and Tscherne (closed).
- *Minor:*
  - *Displacement:* 0–50% displacement
  - *Comminution:* No or minimal comminution
  - *Wound:* No or small open wound (open grade I, closed grade 0)
  - *Energy/fracture pattern:* Low energy/spiral fracture pattern

- *Moderate:*
  - *Displacement:* 51–100% displacement
  - *Comminution:* Minimal comminution, butterfly segment
  - *Wound:* Open grade II, closed grade I
  - *Energy/fracture pattern:* Moderate energy/oblique or transverse fracture pattern
- *Major:*
  - *Displacement:* 100% displacement
  - *Comminution:* Two or more free fragments, segmental fracture
  - *Wound:* Open grades III-IV, closed grades II-III
  - *Energy/fracture pattern:* High, crushing/transverse or fragmented

FOOT AND ANKLE FRACTURES

Lauge-Hansen Classification of Ankle Fractures

- *Supination-Adduction (SA):*
  - Transverse lateral malleolar fracture below the tibial plafond
  - Vertical shearing fracture of the medial malleolus

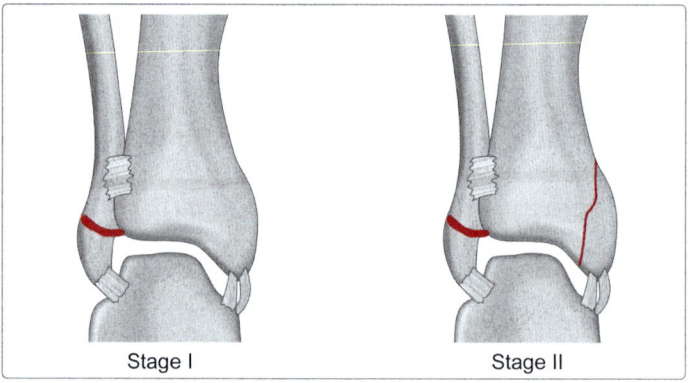

- *Supination external rotation (SER):*
  - Anterior syndesmotic injury
  - Oblique fibular fracture at the level of the plafond

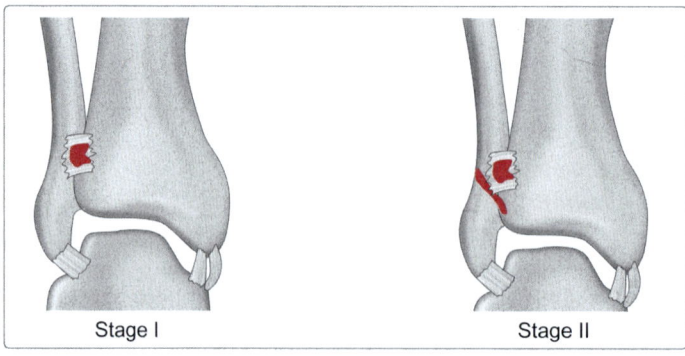

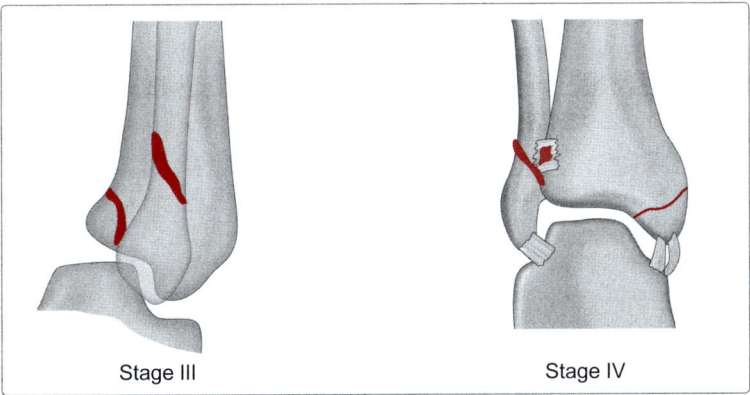

| Stage III | Stage IV |

- Posterior syndesmotic injury and posterior malleolar fracture
- Medial malleolar fracture or deltoid avulsion
○ *Pronation external rotation (PER):*
    - Transverse medial malleolar/deltoid injury
    - Anterior syndesmotic injury
    - Short oblique fracture of fibula above syndesmosis
    - Posterior syndesmosis injury or posterior malleolar fracture

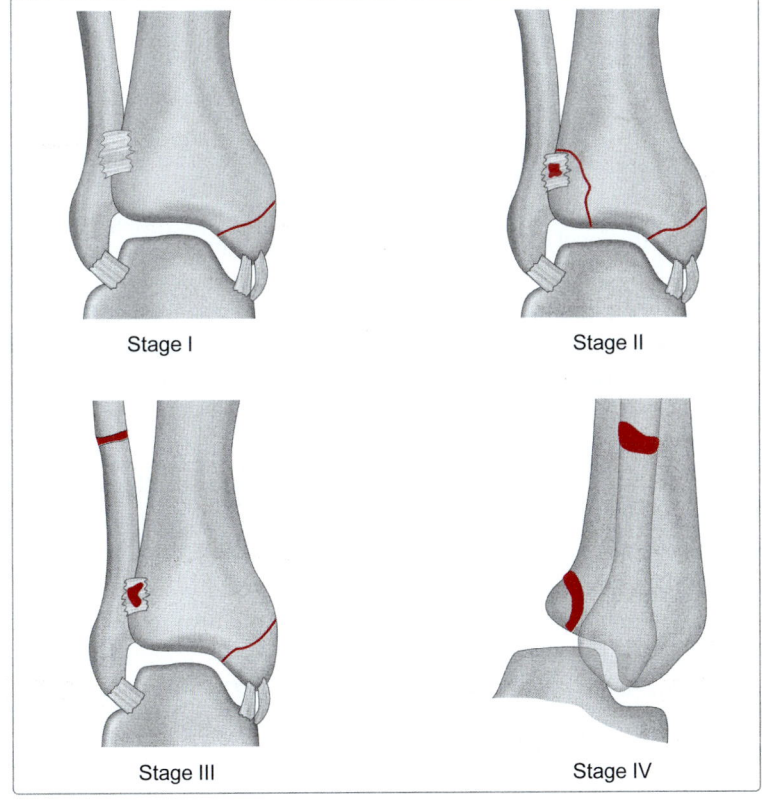

| Stage I | Stage II |
| Stage III | Stage IV |

○ *Pronation-Abduction (PA):*
  - Medial malleolar/deltoid avulsion
  - Syndesmotic injury with interosseous membrane tear
  - High fibular fracture

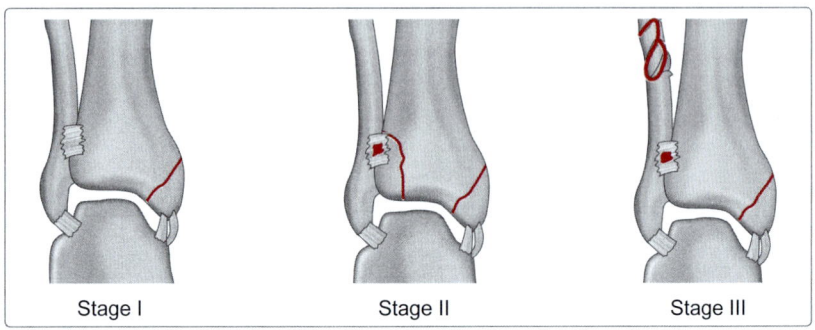

Stage I   Stage II   Stage III

Crude Memorization Technique

○ *If medial malleolus fractured vertically:* SA injury
○ If medial malleolus fractured horizontally → look at lateral malleolus fracture → if below syndesmosis, it is SE injury, if above syndesmosis, it is PA/PE injury (If fibula fracture is comminuted → PA, if transverse → PE)

Danis Weber Classification

○ *Type A:* Describes a fracture of the lateral malleolus distal to the syndesmosis. Usually stable.
  Typical features:
  - Below the level of the tibial plafond (syndesmosis)
  - Tibiofibular syndesmosis intact
  - Deltoid ligament intact
  - Occasional oblique or vertical medial malleolus fracture
○ *Type B:* Describes a fracture at the level of the syndesmosis. Variable stability.
  Typical features:
  - At the level of the ankle joint, extending proximally in an oblique fashion up the fibula
  - Tibiofibular syndesmosis intact or only partially torn, but no widening of the distal tibiofibular articulation
  - Medial malleolus may be fractured or deltoid ligament may be torn.
○ *Type C:* Describes a fracture proximal to the syndesmosis. Unstable requiring open reduction and internal fixation (ORIF).
  Typical features:
  - Above the level of the ankle joint

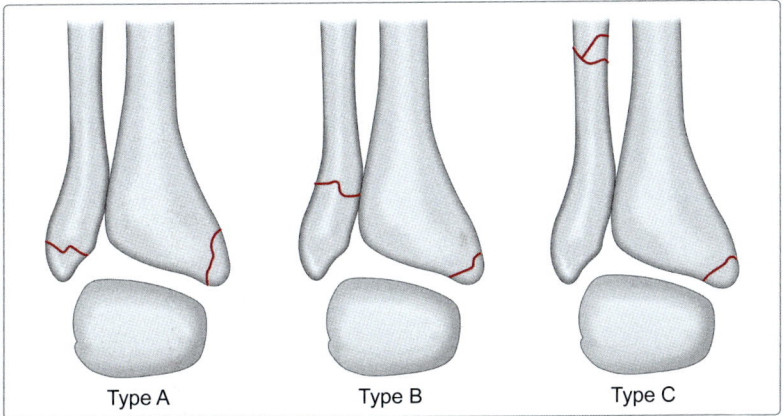

Type A   Type B   Type C

- Tibiofibular syndesmosis injured with widening of the distal tibiofibular articulation
- Medial malleolus fracture or deltoid ligament injury may be present.

TIBIAL PILON FRACTURE

Ruedi and Allgower Classification
- *Type I:* Nondisplaced
- *Type II:* Simple displacement with incongruous joint
- *Type III:* Comminuted articular surface

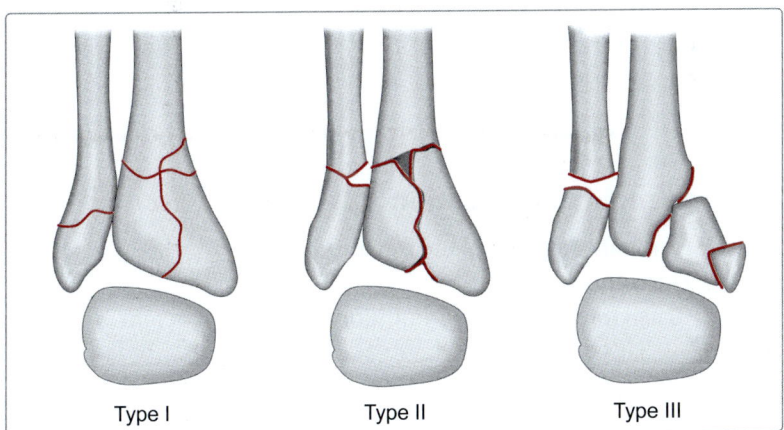

Type I   Type II   Type III

Mast and Pappas Classification
- *Type A:* Fractures with significant posterior lip involvement
- *Type B:* Spiral fracture of distal third tibia with articular extension
- *Type C:* Talar impaction into the articular surface

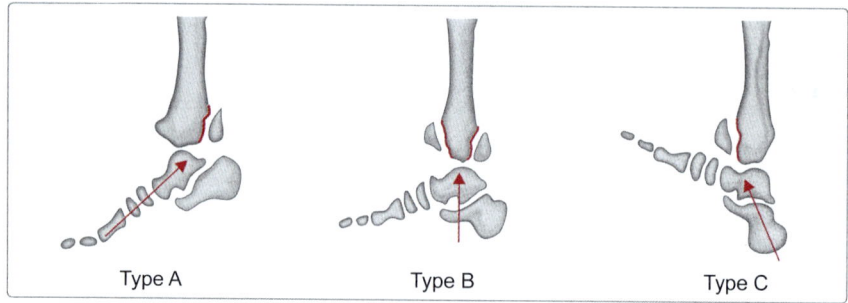

TALAR NECK FRACTURES

Hawkins Classification

- *Type I:* Nondisplaced, 0–13% risk of AVN
- *Type II:* Subtalar dislocation, 20–50% risk of AVN
- *Type III:* Subtalar and tibiotalar dislocation, 20–100% risk of AVN
- *Type IV:* Subtalar, tibiotalar and talonavicular dislocations, 70–100% risk of AVN

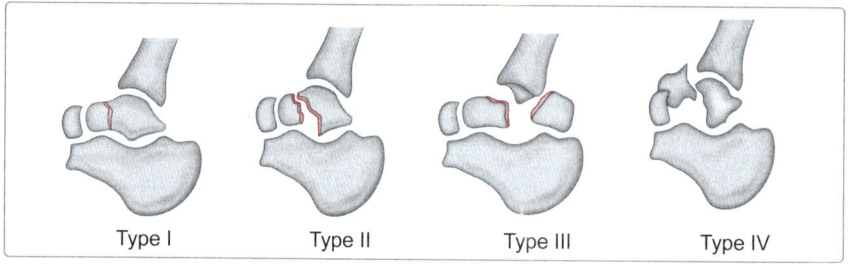

TALAR BODY FRACTURE

Boyd and Knight Classification

- *Type 1:* Coronal or sagittal plane fracture
- *Type 2:* Horizontal fracture
- *Type 3:* Crush fracture with comminution and loss of height

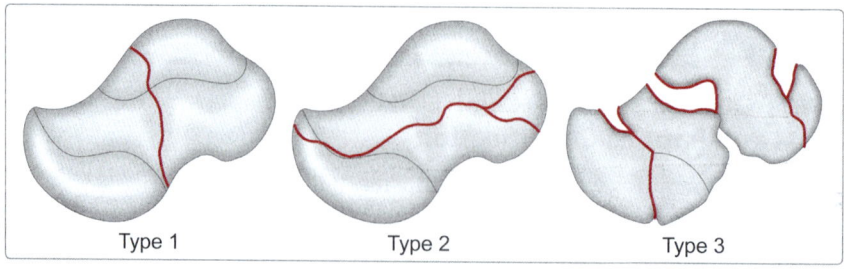

CALCANEUS FRACTURE

Sanders Classification

Based on number of articular fragments seen on coronal CT:
- *Type I:* Nondisplaced
- *Type II:* Two articular fragments (one fracture line in the posterior facet)
- *Type III:* Three articular fragments (two fracture line in the posterior facet)
- *Type IV:* More than three articular fragments (comminuted)

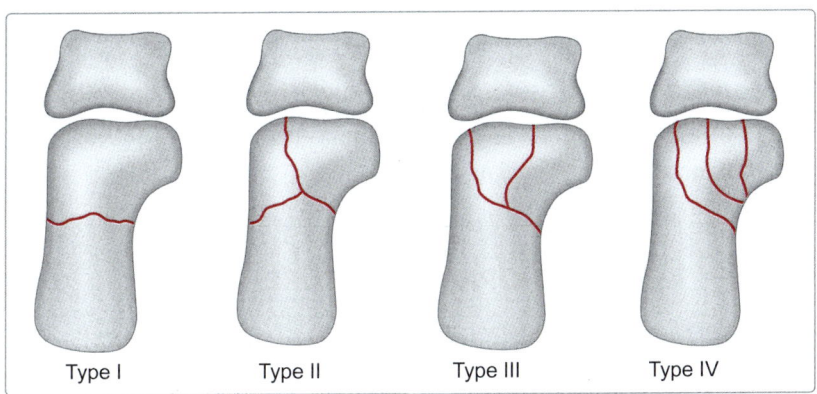

Essex–Lopresti Classification

The *primary fracture* line runs obliquely through the posterior facet forming two fragments.

The *secondary fracture* line runs in one of two planes:
- The axial plane beneath the facet exiting posteriorly in tongue-type fractures
- When the superolateral fragment and posterior facet remain attached to the tuberosity posteriorly
- Behind the posterior facet in joint depression fractures

LISFRANC FRACTURE

Quenu and Kuss Classification

- *Homolateral:* All five metatarsals displaced in the same direction
- *Isolated:* One or two metatarsals displaced from the others
- *Divergent:* Displacement of the metatarsals in both the sagittal and coronal planes

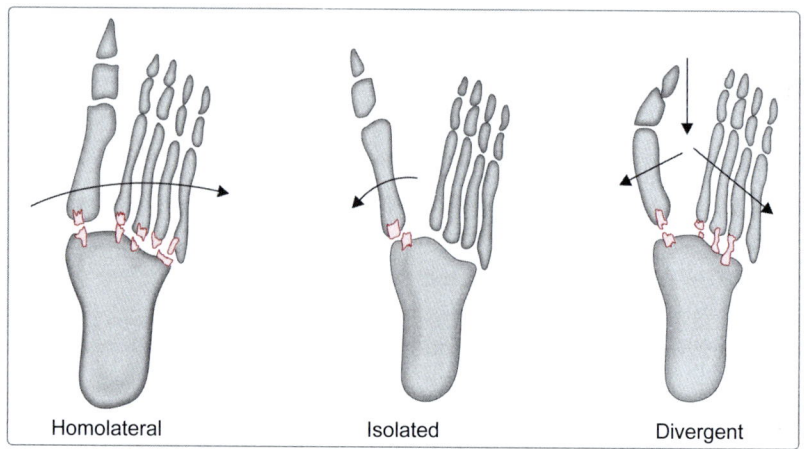

Myerson Classification

- *Total incongruity:* Lateral and dorsoplantar
- *Partial incongruity:* Medial and lateral
- *Divergent:* Partial and total

CHOPART FRACTURE

Main and Jowett Classification

- *Medial stress fracture:* Inversion injury with adduction
- *Longitudinal stress injury:* Fracture of navicular in a vertical pattern
- *Lateral stress injury: Nutcracker fracture* causing crushing of cuboid
- *Plantar stress injury:* Avulsion fracture of the dorsal lip of navicular, talus

NAVICULAR FRACTURE

Sangeorzan's Classification

- *Type I:* Dorsal or tuberosity avulsion fracture, the primary fracture line traverse in the coronal plane.
- *Type II:* Navicular body fracture, in which the fracture line is traverse from dorsolateral to plantarmedial across the body.
- *Type III:* Navicular body fracture with central or lateral comminution.

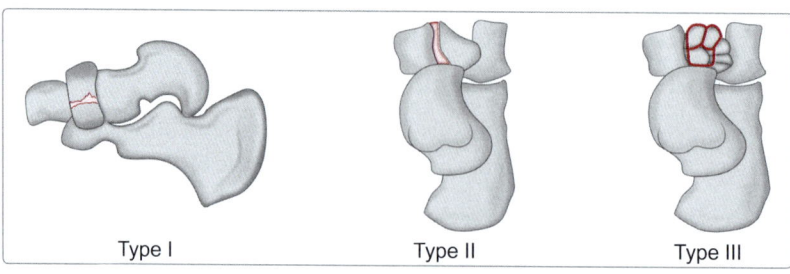

5TH METATARSAL FRACTURE

It is the fracture of the base of the 5th metatarsal.

De Lee Classification

- *Type 1A:* Acute, nondisplaced metadiaphyseal
- *Type 1B:* Acute comminuted metadiaphyseal
- *Type 2:* Chronic metadiaphyseal
- *Type 3A:* Extra-articular styloid avulsion
- *Type 3B:* Intra-articular styloid

Dameron-Lawrence-Bofte Classification

- *Zone 1 fractures:* Associated with inversion injury (avulsion)
- *Zone 2 fractures:* Jones fracture. Indirect forefoot adduction with plantar flexion
- *Zone 3 fractures:* Stress related, repetitive cyclic loading

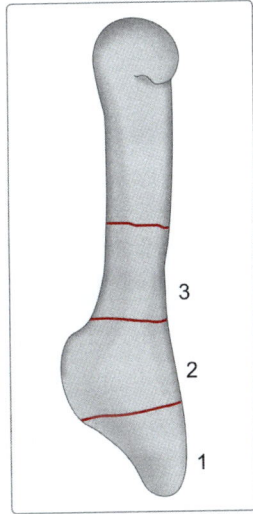

CHAPTER 3

Pediatric Trauma

SALTER–HARRIS PHYSEAL INJURY

- *Type 1:* Fracture through the growth plate (no obvious displacement)
- *Type 2:* Fracture through the growth plate and metaphysis sparing epiphysis (Thurston Holland fragment)
- *Type 3:* Fracture through the growth plate and epiphysis, sparing metaphysis
- *Type 4:* Fracture through the growth plate, metaphysis and epiphysis
- *Type 5:* Late compression fracture of growth plate (very difficult to diagnose)

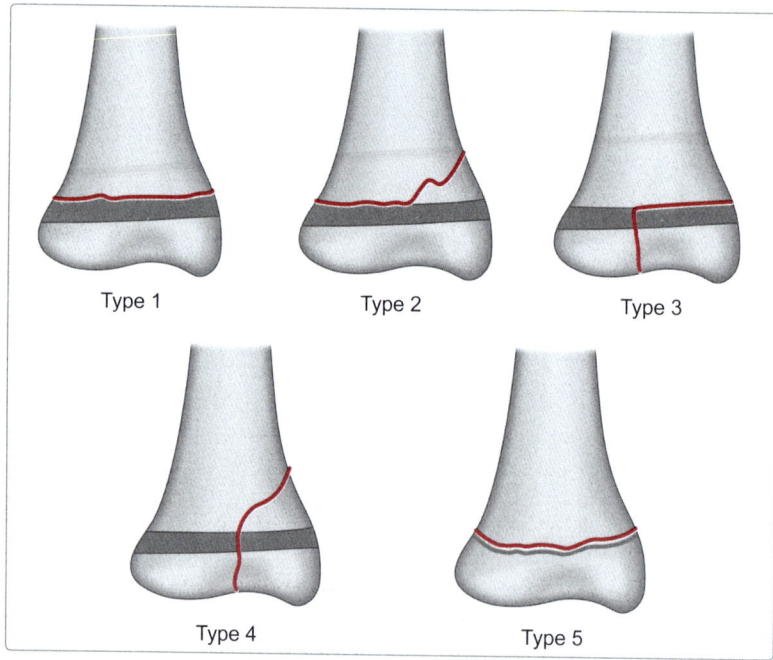

Peterson added two new variants of physeal injuries:
1. *Peterson Type I fracture* is transmetaphyseal with extension into the physis.
2. *Peterson Type VI fracture* has loss of part of the physis and typically is described as an open *"lawnmower"* type of injury.

Ogden Modification to Salter–Harris Classification

- *Type VI:* Injury to the peripheral portion of the physis and a resultant bony bridge formation which may produce an angular deformity
- *Type VII:* Isolated injury of the epiphyseal plate
- *Type VIII:* Isolated injury of the metaphysis with possible impairment of endochondral ossification
- *Type IX:* Injury of the periosteum which may impair intramembranous ossification.

The mnemonic "SALTER" can be used to help remember the first five types:
1. S = Separated or straight across
2. A = Above
3. L = Lower
4. TE = Through Everything
5. R = Rammed (crushed)

PROXIMAL HUMERUS FRACTURE

Neer–Horowitz Classification

- *Grade 1:* Less than 5 mm displacement
- *Grade 2:* Displacement less than one-third the width of the shaft
- *Grade 3:* Displacement one-third to the two-thirds the width of the shaft
- *Grade 4:* Displacement more than two-thirds the width of the shaft, including total displacement.

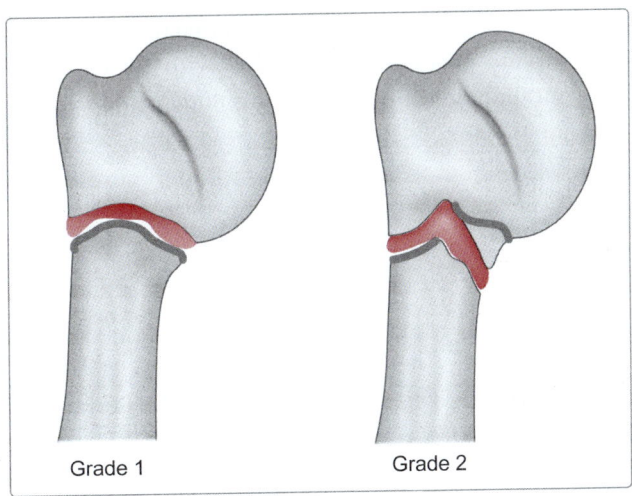

Grade 1 Grade 2

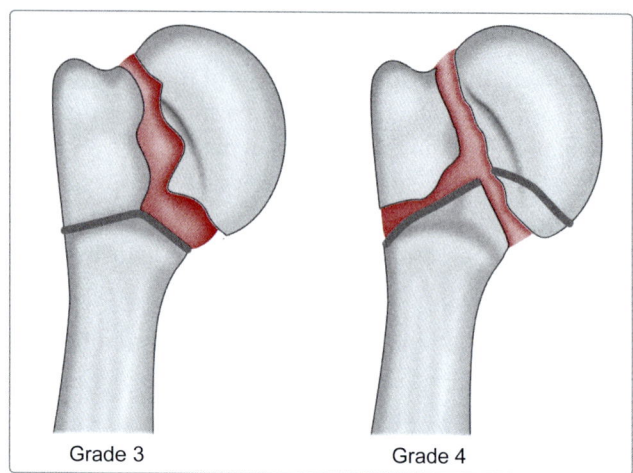

Grade 3   Grade 4

Note: Acceptable angulation—proximal humerus and shaft in humerus fracture.

- *<5 years:* 70° angulation and 100% displacement
- *5–11 years:* 40–70° of angulation
- *>11 years:* <40° angulation and <50% displacement
- *Age 12 years to maturity:* 15–20° of angulation and displacement of <30% the width of the shaft

SUPRACONDYLAR ELBOW FRACTURE

Gartland Classification

- *Type 1:* Nondisplaced
- *Type 2:* Displaced with intact posterior cortex, may be slightly angulated or rotated
- *Type 3:* Complete displacement; posteromedial or posterolateral
- *Type 4:* Complete periosteal disruption with flexion and extension instability (intraoperative finding, recently added type).

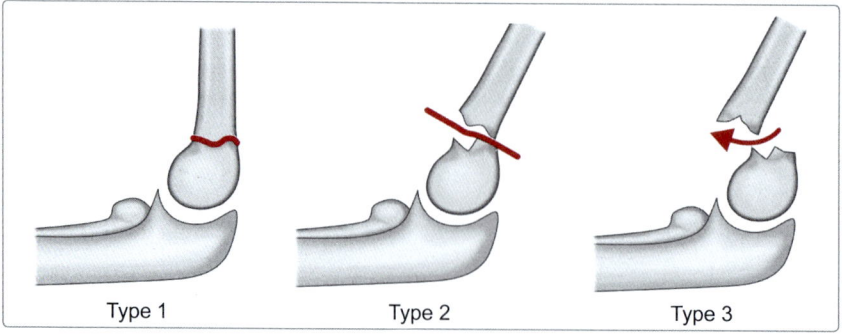

Type 1   Type 2   Type 3

LATERAL CONDYLE HUMERUS PHYSEAL FRACTURES

Milch Classification

- *Type 1 (less common):* Fracture line courses lateral to the trochlea and into the capitulotrochlear groove (Salter–Harris type 4 fracture).
- *Type 2 (more common and severe):* Fracture line extends into the apex of the trochlea, (Salter–Harris type 2 fracture).

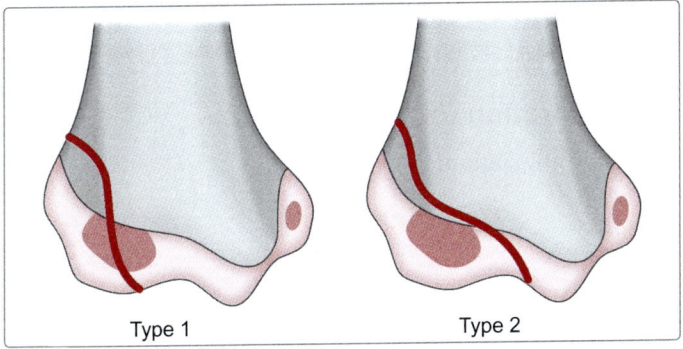

Jakob Classification

- *Stage 1:* Nondisplaced fracture or minimally displaced fracture (<3 mm)
- *Stage 2:* Complete fracture with moderate displacement (>3 mm)
- *Stage 3:* Complete displacement and rotation

MEDIAL CONDYLE HUMERUS PHYSEAL FRACTURES

Milch Classification

- *Type 1 (more common):* Fracture line transverses through the apex of the trochlea (Salter–Harris type 2 fracture).
- *Type 2 (less common):* Fracture line through capitulotrochlear groove (Salter–Harris type 4 fracture).

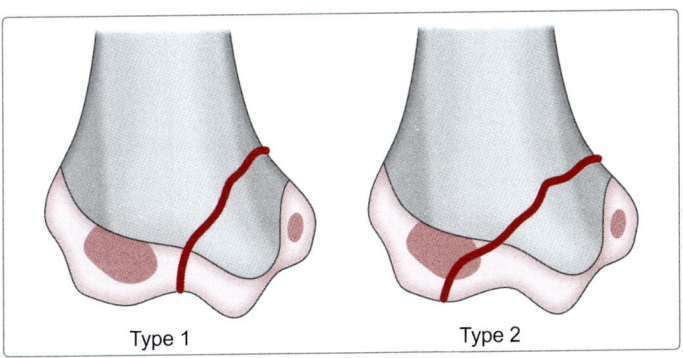

Pediatric Trauma

ACCEPTABLE ALIGNMENT DURING EARLY PHASES OF BOTH BONE FOREARM FRACTURE			
Age	**Angulation**	**Malrotation degree**	**Displacement**
0–10 years	<15	<45	yes if <1 cm
>10 years	<10	<30	No
Approaching skeletal maturity (<2 years growth left)	0	0	No

RADIAL HEAD AND NECK FRACTURES

O'Brien Classification

Based on fracture angulation:
- *Type 1:* 0–30°
- *Type 2:* 30–60°
- *Type 3:* >60°

Wilkins Classification

- *Type 1:* Salter–Harris type 1 or 2 physeal injury
- *Type 2:* Salter–Harris type 3 or 4 intra-articular injury
- *Type 3:* Fracture line completely within metaphysis
- *Type 4:* Fractures occurring when a dislocated elbow is being reduced
- *Type 5:* Fractures occurring in conjunction with the elbow dislocation

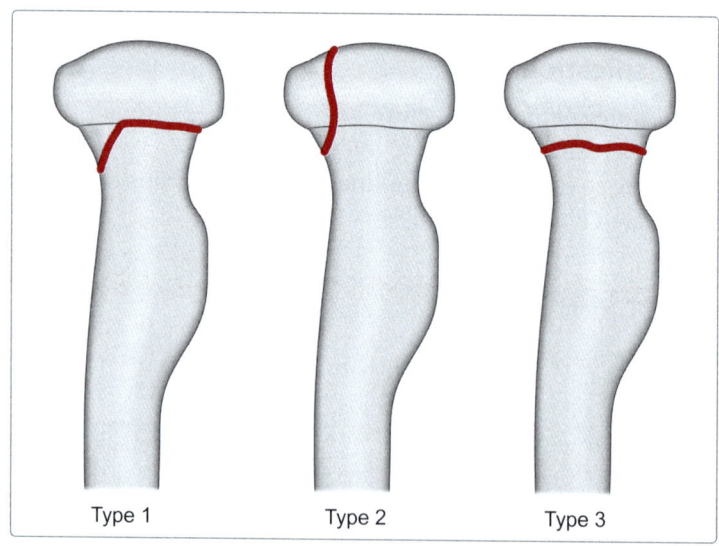

PEDIATRIC PELVIC FRACTURE

Torode and Zieg Classification

- Avulsion fractures
- Iliac wing fractures:
  - Separation of the iliac apophysis
  - Fracture of the bony iliac wing
- Simple ring fractures:
  - Fractures of the pubic and disruption of the pubic symphysis
  - Fractures involving the acetabulum, without a concomitant ring fractures
- Fractures producing an unstable segment:
  - Straddle fractures, characterized by bilateral inferior and superior pubic rami fracture
  - Fractures involving the anterior pubic rami or pubic symphysis and the posterior elements
  - Fractures that create an unstable segment between the anterior ring of the pelvis and the acetabulum

FRACTURES OF THE NECK OF FEMUR

Delbet Classification

- *Type 1:* Transepiphyseal fracture (osteonecrosis approaches 100%)
- *Type 2:* Transcervical fractures (most common type) (osteonecrosis approaches 50%)

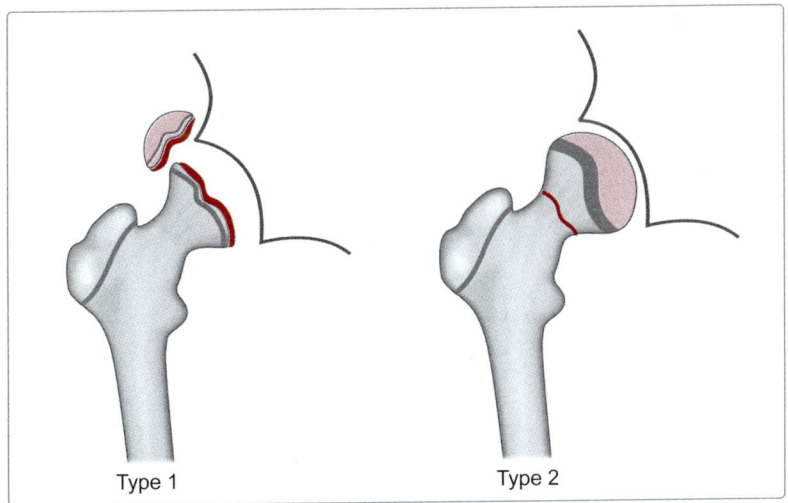

- *Type 3:* Cervicotrochanteric fracture (osteonecrosis approaches 20–30%)
- *Type 4:* Intertrochanteric fracture

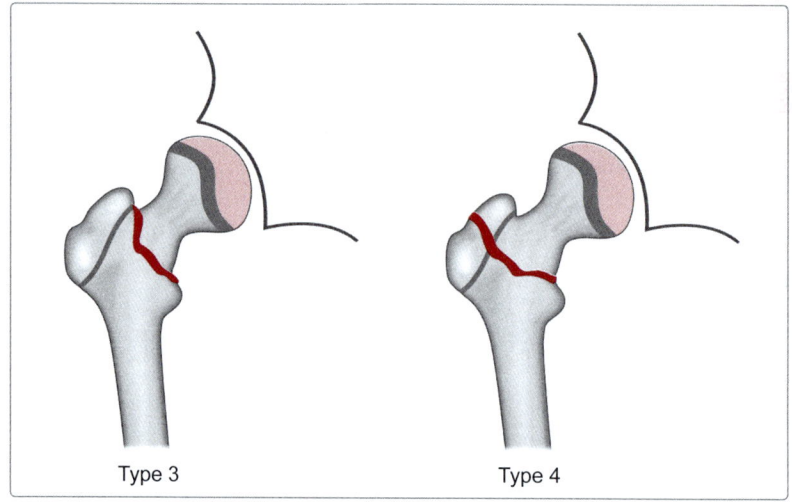

TIBIAL TUBERCLE FRACTURES

Watson and Jones Classification
- *Type 1:* Small fragment avulsed and displaced proximally
- *Type 2:* Secondary ossification center already coalesced with proximal tibial epiphysis; fracture at junction
- *Type 3:* Fracture line passing proximally through the tibial epiphysis and into joint.

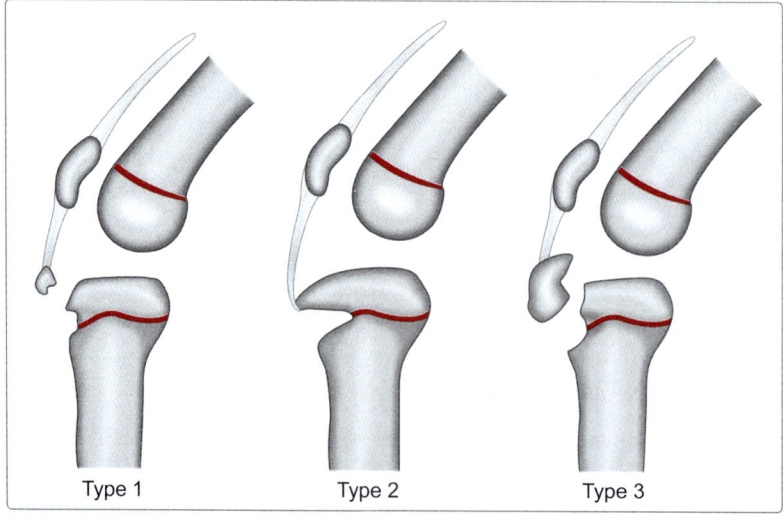

CHAPTER 4

Spine Trauma

SPINAL CORD INJURY

Modified Frankel Classification

- *Grade A:* Absent motor and sensory
- *Grade B:* Absent motor function; sensory present
- *Grade C:* Motor function present but not useful (2/5 or 3/5); sensation present (non-functional for any useful purpose)
- *Grade D1:* Preserved motor at lowest functional grade (3+ to 5+) and/or with bowel or bladder paralysis with normal or reduced voluntary motor function
- *Grade D2:* Preserved motor at mid functional grade (3+ to 4+/5+) and/or with neurogenic bowel or bladder dysfunction
- *Grade D3:* Preserved at high functional grade (4+ to 5+) and normal voluntary bowel or bladder function
- *Grade E:* Normal motor (5/5); and sensory function

AMERICAN SPINAL INJURY ASSOCIATION (ASIA) IMPAIRMENT SCALE

- *Grade A:* Complete, no motor sensory function preserved in sacral segments S4–5
- *Grade B:* Incomplete sensory but no motor function preserved below the neurogenic level and extending through the sacral segments S4–5
- *Grade C:* Incomplete motor function preserved below the neurogenic level; most key muscles below the neurogenic level have muscle grade <3
- *Grade D:* Incomplete motor function preserved below the neurogenic level have a muscle grade >3
- *Grade E:* Normal motor and sensory function normal

OCCIPITAL CONDYLE FRACTURE

Anderson and Montesano Classification

- *Type 1:* Impaction of the condyle due to occipital loading
- *Type 2:* Basilar or skull fractures that extend into the condyles
- *Type 3:* Avulsion of the condyle due excessive loading in rotation or lateral rotation or lateral bending (unstable).

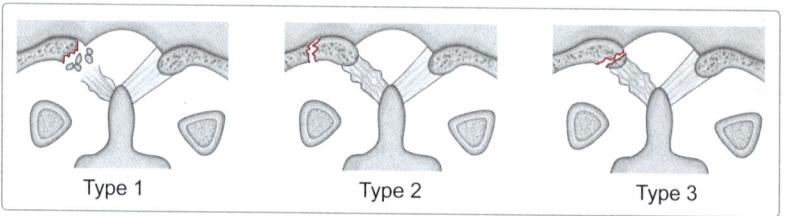

ATLANTO-OCCIPITAL DISLOCATION

Traynelis Classification

- *Type 1:* Occipital condyles anterior to the atlas; most common
- *Type 2:* Condyles longitudinally dissociated from atlas without translation; result of pure distraction
- *Type 3:* Occipital condyles posterior to the atlas

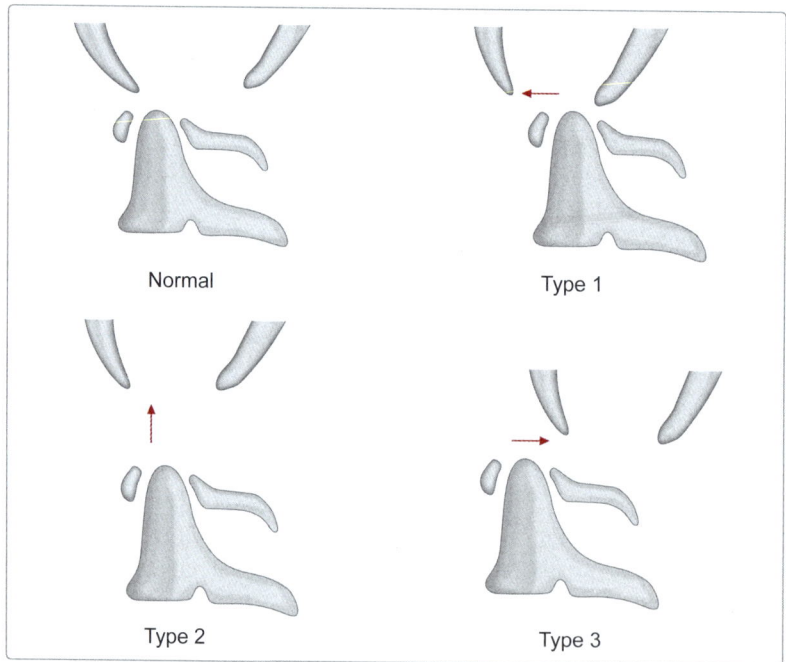

ATLAS FRACTURE (JEFFERSON'S FRACTURE)

Levine and Edwards Classification

Three primary types of fractures of the ring of the C1 have been identified:
1. *Posterior arch fracture:* It usually occurs at the junction of the posterior arch and the lateral mass.

2. *Lateral mass fracture:* It usually occurs on one side only with the fracture line passing either through the articular surface or just anterior and posterior to the lateral mass on one side.
3. *Burst fracture (Jefferson's fracture):* It is characterized by four fractures. Two in the posterior arch and two in the anterior arch.

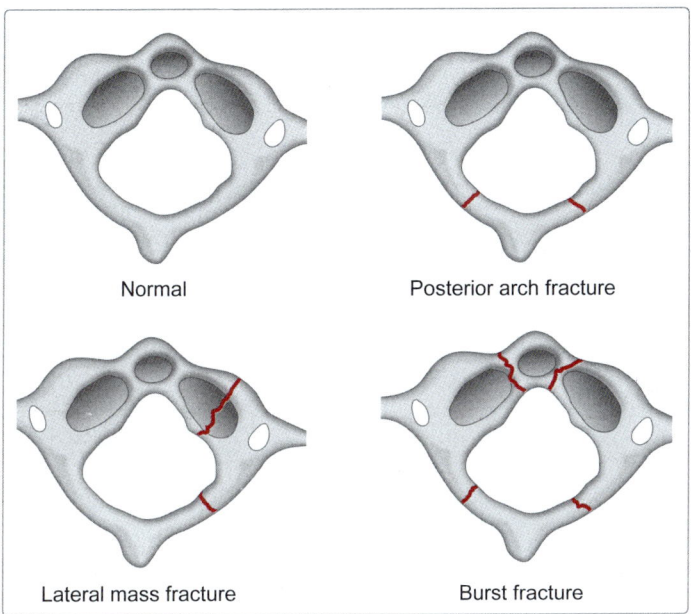

ATLANTOAXIAL ROTATORY SUBLUXATION AND DISLOCATION

Fielding and Hawkins Classification

- *Type 1:* Odontoid as a pivot point; no neurological injury, atlanto-dental interval (ADI) < 3 mm; transverse ligament intact
- *Type 2:* Opposite facet as a pivot; ADI 3–5 mm; transverse ligament insufficient
- *Type 3:* Both joints anteriorly subluxated; ADI > 5 mm; transverse and alar ligaments incompetent
- *Type 4:* Rare, both joints posteriorly subluxed
- *Type 5:* Frank dislocation

FRACTURES OF THE ODONTOID PROCESS (DENS)

Anderson and D'Alonzo Classification

- *Type 1:* Oblique avulsion fracture of the apex

- *Type 2:* Fracture at the junction of the body and the neck; high nonunion rates:
  - *Type 2A:* With comminution
  - *Type 2B:* Without comminution
- *Type 3:* Fracture extends into the body of the C-2 and may involve the lateral facets.

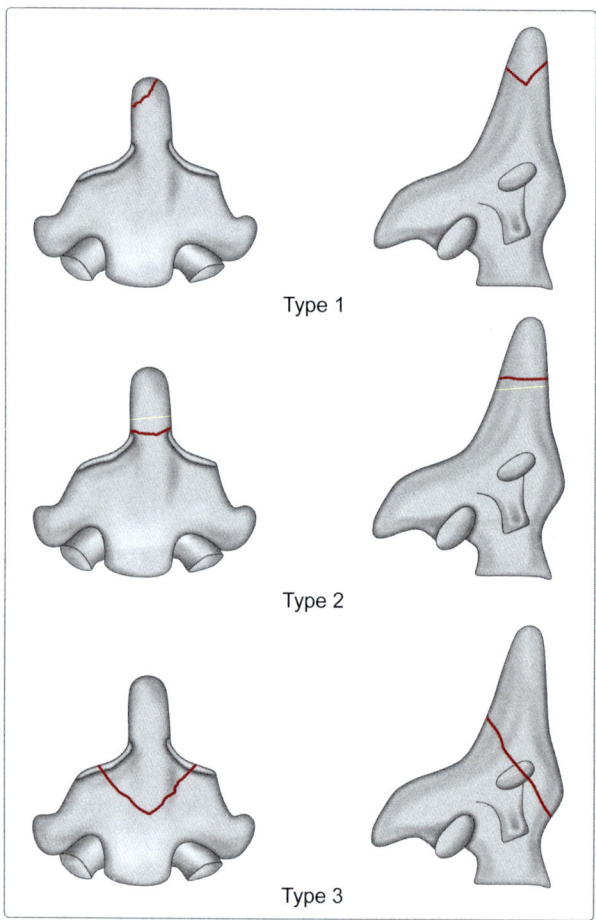

TRAUMATIC SPONDYLOLISTHESIS OF C-2 (HANGMAN'S FRACTURE)

Levine and Edwards Classification

- *Type 1:* Nondisplaced, no angulation; no translation <3 mm; stable; C2-3 disk intact
- *Type 2:* Significant angulation at C2-3; translation >3 mm; most common injury pattern; unstable; C2-3 disk disrupted

- *Type 2A:* Minimal translation, but significant angulation; Avulsion of the entire C2–3 intervertebral disk in flexion, leaving the anterior longitudinal ligament intact
- *Type 3:* Results from initial anterior facet dislocation of C2 on C3 followed by extension injury fracturing the neural arch.

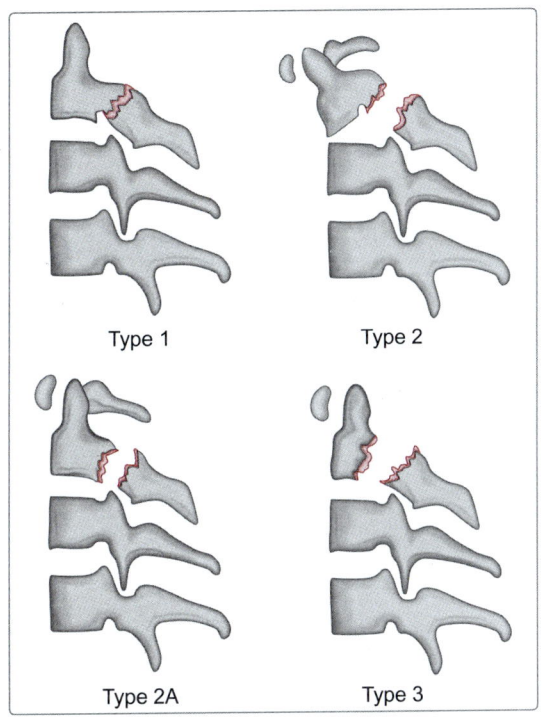

THORACOLUMBAR FRACTURES

McAfee Classification

- Wedge compression fracture
- Unstable burst fracture
- Flexion distraction injury
- Stable burst fracture
- Chance fracture
- Translation fracture

THORACOLUMBAR INJURY CLASSIFICATION AND SEVERITY SCORE OF VACCARO (TLICSS)	
Fracture morphology/mechanism	*Points*
Compression	1
Lateral angulation >15°	1
Burst	1
Translation/rotational	3
Distraction	4

Contd...

Contd...

Neurologic involvement	Points
Intact	0
Nerve root	2
Cord, conus medullaris: • Incomplete • Complete	3 2
Cauda equina	3
Posterior ligamentous complex status	
Intact	0
Injury suspected/intermediate	2
Injured	3

SACRAL FRACTURES

Denis Classification

- *Type 1:* Region of ala (5.9% risk of neurological injury)
- *Type 2:* Region of sacral foramina (30% risk of neurological injury)
- *Type 3:* Region of central canal

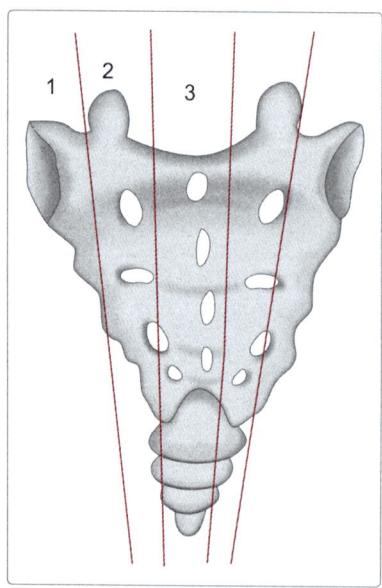

CHAPTER 5

Upper Limb Regional Conditions

FROZEN SHOULDER

Primary frozen shoulder has three phases:
- *Phase 1:* Characterized by pain (freezing phase)
- *Phase 2:* Characterized by stiffness (frozen phase); Scapulothoracic symptoms predominate in this phase due to compensatory mechanisms.
- *Phase 3:* Thawing

Arthroscopic Staging
- *Stage 1:* Preadhesive, full motion with pain especially at night
- *Stage 2:* Acute adhesive synovitis, mild restriction of movements and pain as predominant feature
- *Stage 3:* Maturation—motion significantly restricted with less severe pain
- *Stage 4:* Chronic; severe painless restriction of movements

IMPINGEMENT SYNDROME

- *Stage 1:* Reversible edema and hemorrhage are present in a patient under age of 25 years.
- *Stage 2:* Fibrosis and tendonitis affect the rotator cuff of a patient typically 25–40 years of age.
- *Stage 3:* Bone spurs and tendon ruptures are present in a patient over the age of 40 years.

CALCIFIC TENDINITIS

The following three-phase chronology is described by *Sarkar and Uhthoff:*
- *Phase 1—Precalcification stage:* Here the chondrocytes mediate the calcium deposition at multiple foci
- *Phase 2—Calcific stage:*
  - *Phase of formation:* Phagocytic cells accumulate and vascular proliferation takes place.
  - *Phase of resorption:* The resorptive phase begins when these vascular channels provide a pathway for resorption and restore normal tension and perfusion to these tissues.
- *Phase 3:* Postcalcific phase

SUPERIOR LABRUM ANTERIOR AND POSTERIOR (SLAP) TEAR

Snyder Classification

- *Type 1:*
  - Fraying and degeneration of the superior labrum, normal biceps
  - Most common type of SLAP tears (75% of SLAP tears)
  - These are treated with debridement.
- *Type 2:*
  - Detachment of superior labrum and biceps insertion from the supraglenoid tubercle
  - May resemble a normal variant (Buford complex)
  - *Three subtypes:* Based on detachment of labrum involved (anterior aspect of labrum alone, the posterior aspect alone, or both aspects)
  - Treatment involves anatomic arthroscopic repair.

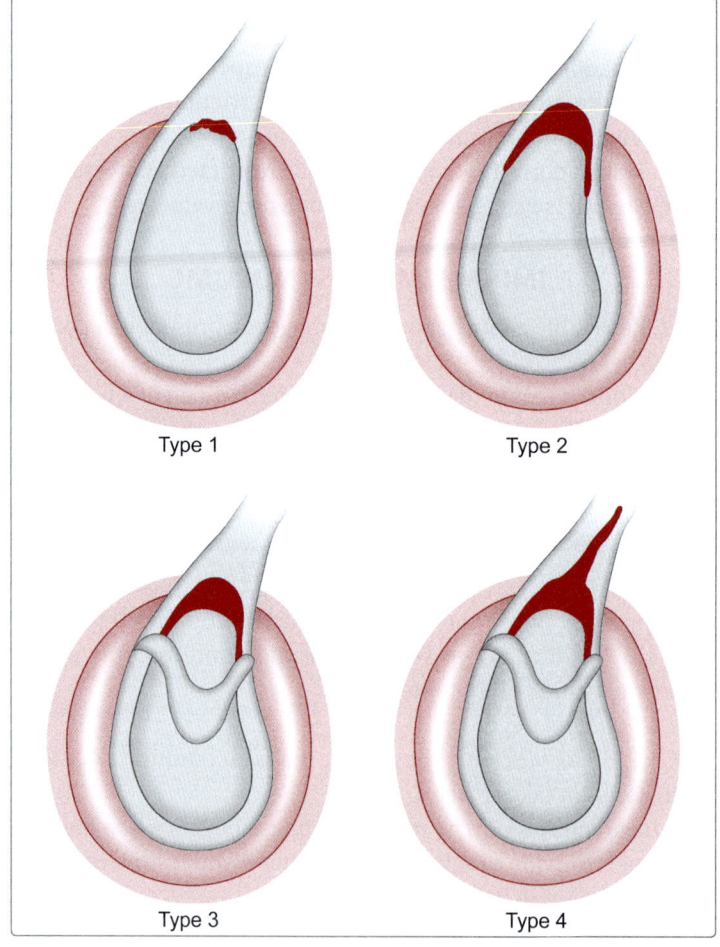

- *Type 3:*
    - Bucket handle type tear
    - Biceps anchor is intact
    - *Treatment:* Debride labrum
- *Type 4:*
    - Vertical tear of the superior labrum, which extends into biceps.
    - May be treated with repair of labrum and biceps tear.

DUPUYTREN'S CONTRACTURE

- *Grade 1* disease presents as a thickened nodule and a band in the palmar aponeurosis; this band may progress to skin tethering, puckering, or pitting.
- *Grade 2* presents as a peritendinous band, and extension of the affected finger is limited.
- *Grade 3* presents as flexion contracture.

TRIGGER FINGER

Eastwood Classification

- *Grade 0:* Involving mild crepitus in a nontriggering digit
- *Grade 1:* Uneven movement of the digit
- *Grade 2:* Clicking without locking
- *Grade 3:* Locking of the digit that is either actively or passively correctable
- *Grade 4:* A locked digit

BRACHIAL PLEXUS INJURY

Leffert Classification

- *I:* Open (usually from stabbing)
- *II:* Closed (usually from motorcycle accident)
- *IIa:* Supraclavicular

Preganglionic:
- Avulsion of nerve roots, usually from high velocity injuries
- No proximal stump, no neuroma formation (negative Tinel's sign)
- Pseudomeningocele, denervation of rhomboids and serratus anterior
- Horner's sign (ptosis, miosis, anhidrosis, enophthalmos, loss of ciliospinal reflex)
- Normal histamine test (C8-T1 sympathetic ganglion) intact triple response (redness, wheal, flare)
- Elevated hemidiaphragm (phrenic nerve involvement)

Postganglionic:
- Roots remain intact
- Usually from traction injuries
- Proximal stump remains and neuroma formation (positive Tinel's sign)
- Rhomboids and serratus anterior are intact.
- Pseudomeningoceles will not develop.

Infraclavicular lesion: Usually involves branches from the trunks (supraclavicular)
- *III:* Radiation induced
- *IV:* Obstetric
- *IVa:* Erb's (upper root)—Waiter's tip/Porter's tip hand
- *IVb:* Klumpke (lower root)

Classification as Per Site

- Root
- Trunk
- Cord
- Divisions

Relation to Clavicle

- Supraclavicular
- Retroclavicular
- Infraclavicular

ROTATOR CUFF TEARS

Cofield Classification of Rotator Cuff Tears

- *Small:* < 1 cm
- *Medium:* 1–3 cm
- *Large:* 3–5 cm
- *Massive:* > 5 cm

Complete Cuff Tears: Bateman Classification

- *Grade 1:* Tear < 1 cm after debridement
- *Grade 2:* Tear 1–3 cm after debridement
- *Grade 3:* <5 cm
- *Grade 4:* Global tear, no cuff left

Partial Thickness Rotator Cuff Tears: Arthroscopic Classification by Ellman

- *Grade 1:* Partial tear < 3 mm deep
- *Grade 2:* Partial tear 3–6 mm deep (depth not exceeding one-half of the tendon thickness)
- *Grade 3:* Partial tear > 6 mm deep

ELBOW INSTABILITY

- *Valgus posterolateral rotatory:* Seen after simple or complex elbow dislocations.
  - *Simple:* Capsuloligamentous injury without fractures
  - *Complex:* Capsuloligamentous injury with concurrent fracture(s) of radial head fracture/coronoid fracture.
  - *Terrible triad*: Elbow dislocation with associated radial head and coronoid process fracture.

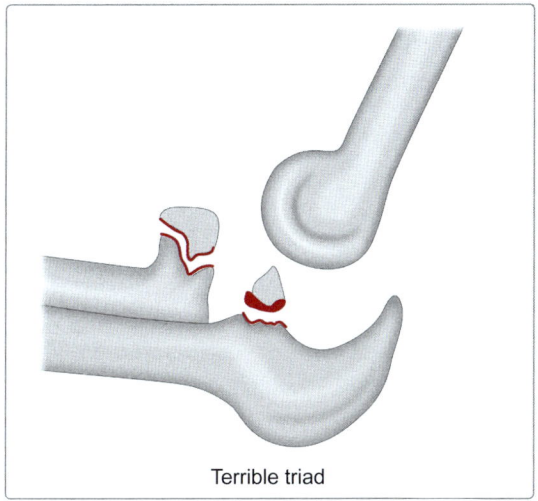

Terrible triad

- Varus posteromedial rotatory instability involves anteromedial coronoid facet fractures and typically results from a subluxation rather than a dislocation.
- *Olecranon fractures:* May be anterior or posterior.

O'Driscoll Classification

- *Timing:* Acute, chronic, recurrent
- *Articulations involved:*
  - The hinge joint (humerus, radius, and ulna)
  - The proximal radioulnar joint
  - Combination
- *Direction of displacement:*
  - Posterolateral rotatory instability
  - Anterior
  - Valgus
  - Varus
- Degree of displacement/soft tissue injury

SCAPHOID LUNATE ADVANCED COLLAPSE (SLAC)

Watson Classification

- *Stage I:* Osteoarthritis of the articulation between the radial styloid and the scaphoid
- *Stage II:* Osteoarthritis involving the whole radioscaphoid articulation
- *Stage III:* Osteoarthritis of the radioscaphoid and capitolunate articulations
- *Stage IV:* Osteoarthritis of the radiocarpal and intercarpal articulations ± distal radioulnar joint (DRUJ)

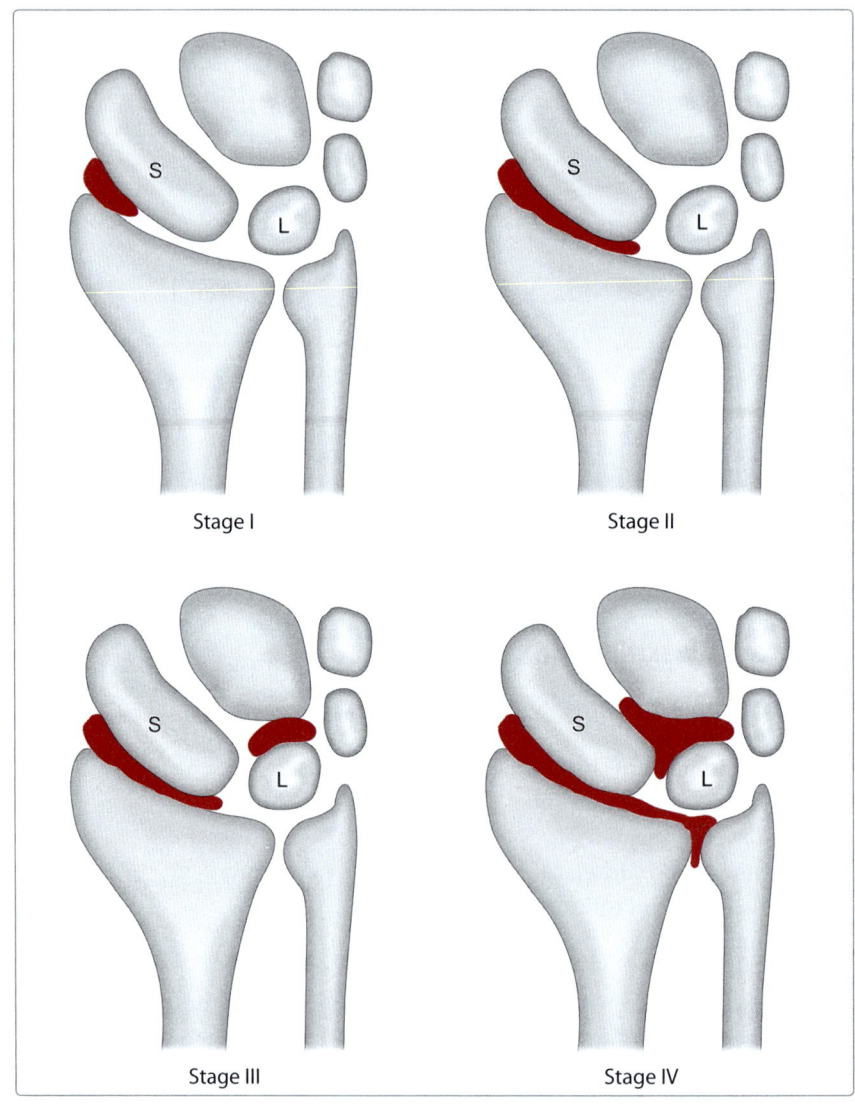

PERILUNATE DISLOCATION

Mayfield Classification
- *Stage I:* Scapholunate dissociation (rotatory subluxation of the scaphoid)
- *Stage II:* Perilunate dislocation
- *Stage III:* Midcarpal dislocation
- *Stage IV:* Lunate dislocation

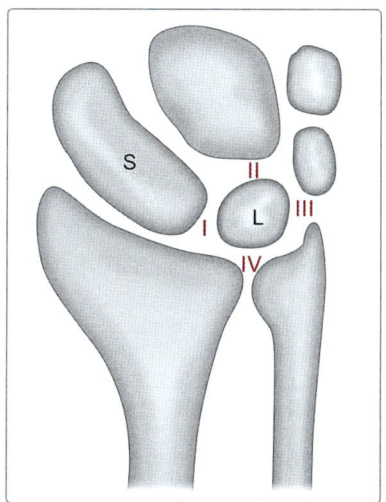

KIENBOCK'S DISEASE

Lichtman Classification
- *Stage 1:* No visible changes on radiograph, but changes seen in MRI
- *Stage 2:* Sclerosis of lunate

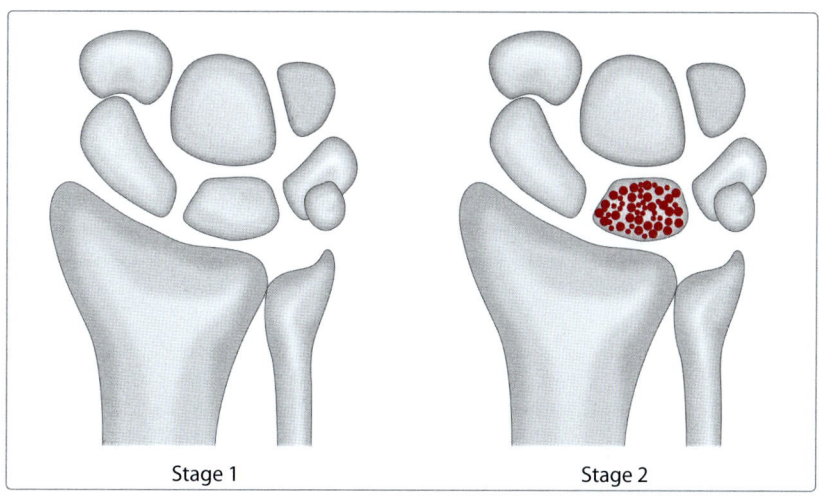

- *Stage 3:* Fragmentation of lunate, without scaphoid rotation
- *Stage 4:* Fragmentation of lunate with fixed rotation of scaphoid

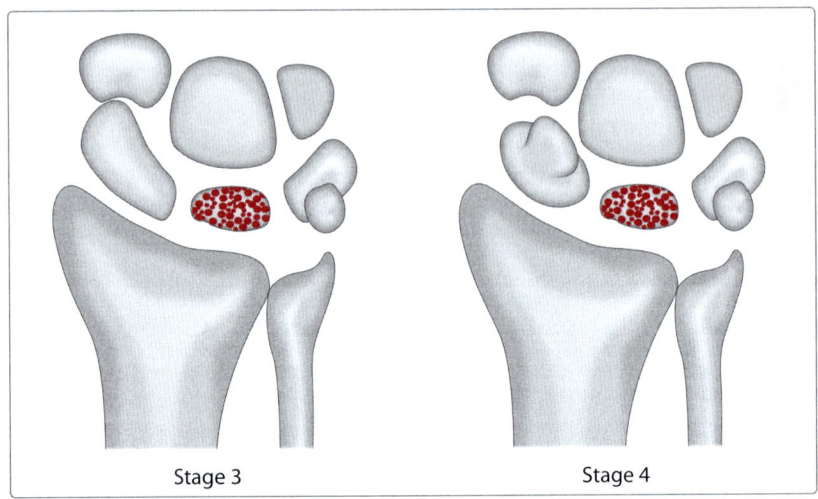

Stage 3   Stage 4

REFLEX SYMPATHETIC DYSTROPHY (RSD)

- *Type I:* RSD/Sudeck's atrophy/algoneurodystrophy
  - Tissue damage with no demonstrable nerve lesions. It is the most common type.
- *Type II:* Causalgia
  - Tissue damage with evidence of nerve damage present.

CHAPTER 6

Lower Limb Regional Conditions

PERTHES DISEASE

Salter-Thompson Classification

- *Group A:* It includes Catterall groups I and II, where the crescent sign involves less than 50% of the femoral head.
- *Group B:* It includes Catterall groups III and IV, where the crescent sign involves more than 50% of the femoral head.

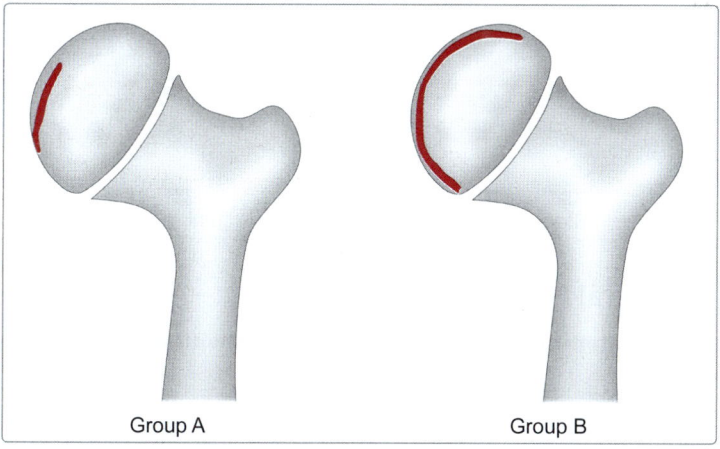

Group A   Group B

Catterall Classification

- *Stage I:* Bone resorption changes visible in the anterior aspect of the epiphysis of femoral head, changes are visible best in frog leg lateral view, no sclerosis is seen.
- *Stage II:* Further bone resorption with slight femoral head collapse in the anterior aspect of femoral head, sclerosis seen.
- *Stage III:* Almost entire femoral head involved in collapse with characteristic head within head appearance, sclerosis seen.
- *Stage IV:* Complete collapse of femoral head with flattening and formation of dense sclerosis; additional metaphyseal changes may be visible, sclerosis seen, posterior remodeling.

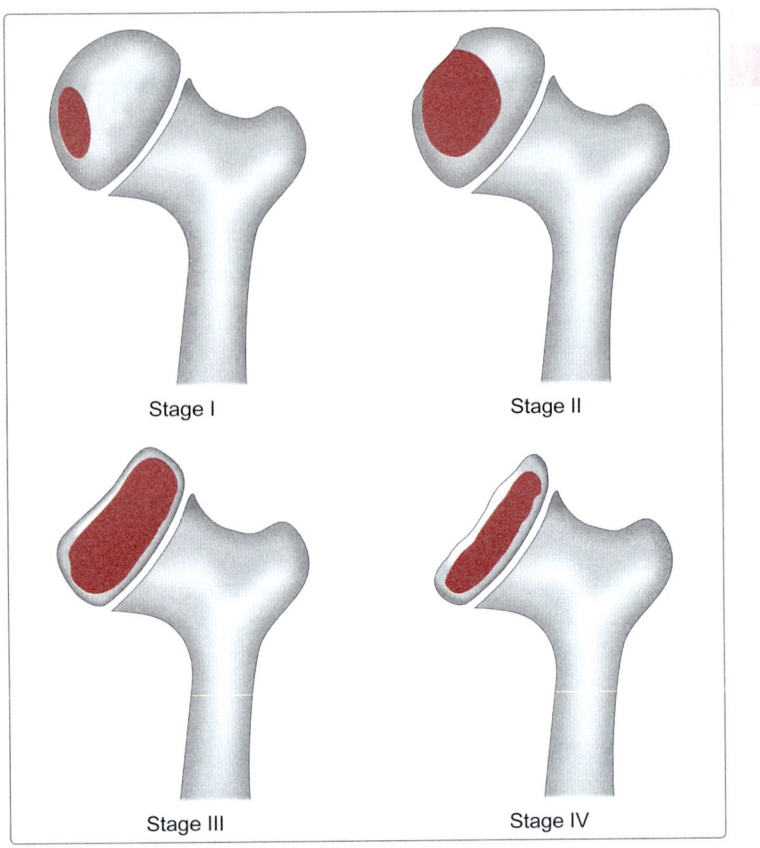

Herring Lateral Pillar Classification

- *Group A:* Lateral pillar maintains full height with no density changes identified.
- *Group B:* Maintains >50% height.
- *Group C:* Less than 50% of lateral pillar height is maintained.

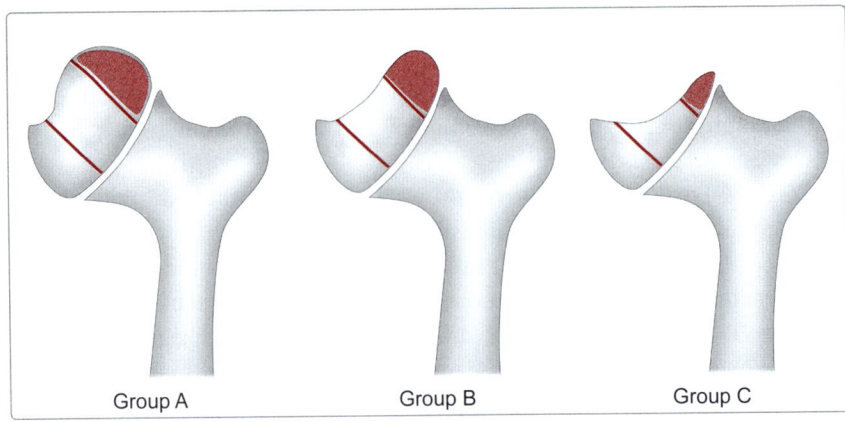

Stulberg Classification

STULBERG CLASSIFICATION			
Class	Description	Radiologic aspect	Prognosis
I	Spherical congruency	Normal	Good
II	Spherical congruency Loss of head shape <2 mm	*Spherical head with one or more of the following findings:* Coxa magna, short femoral neck, upriding greater trochanter, oblique acetabulum	Good
III	Aspherical congruency Loss of head shape >2 mm	Non-spherical head but not flat	Mild-to-moderate arthritis
IV	Aspherical congruency	Flat head and acetabulum	*Poor:* Moderate arthritis
V	Aspherical incongruency	Flat head Normal neck and acetabulum	*Bad:* Severe early arthritis

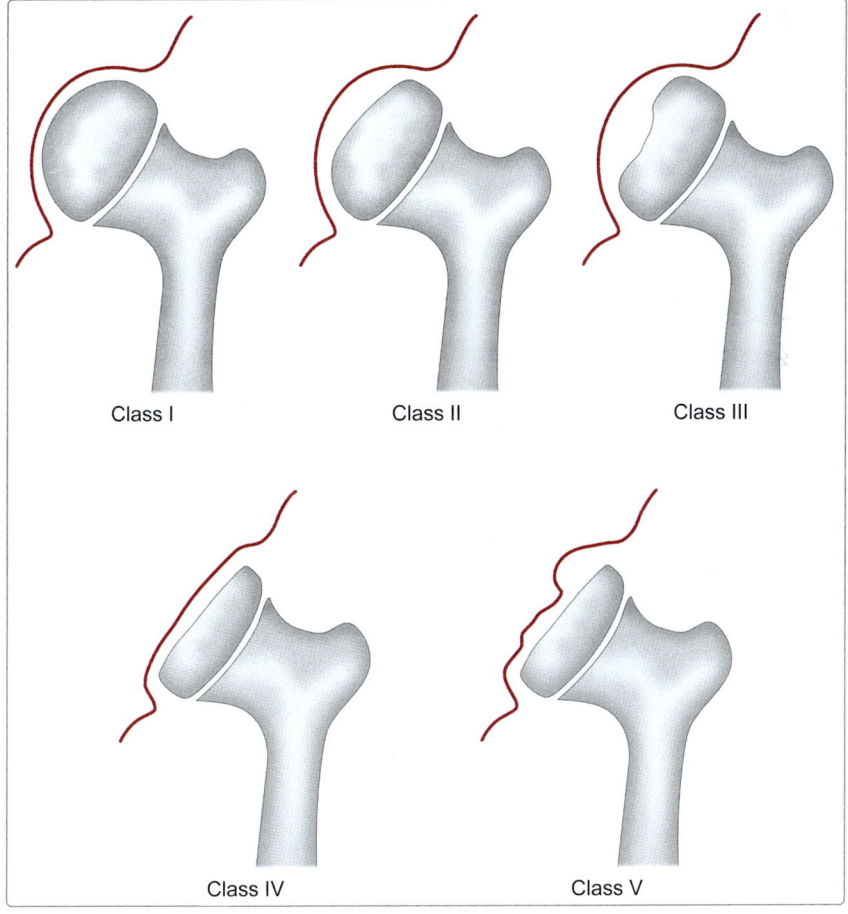

Class I   Class II   Class III

Class IV   Class V

Elizabethtown Classification

I. *Sclerotic:*
   - *Stage Ia:* Part or whole of the epiphysis is sclerotic. There is no loss of height of the epiphysis.
   - *Stage Ib:* The epiphysis is sclerotic and there is loss of epiphyseal height. There is no evidence of fragmentation of the epiphysis.

II. *Fragmentation:*
   - *Stage IIa:* The sclerotic epiphysis has just begun to fragment. One or two vertical fissures are seen in either the anteroposterior (AP) or the lateral views.
   - *Stage IIb:* Fragmentation is advanced. No new bone is visible lateral to the fragmented epiphysis.

III. *Healing:*
   - *Stage IIIa:* Early new bone formation is visible on the periphery of the necrotic epiphysis. The texture of the new bone is not normal; it is "porotic" and covers less than a third of the width of the epiphysis.
   - *Stage IIIb:* The new bone is of normal texture and has grown over a third of the width of the epiphysis.

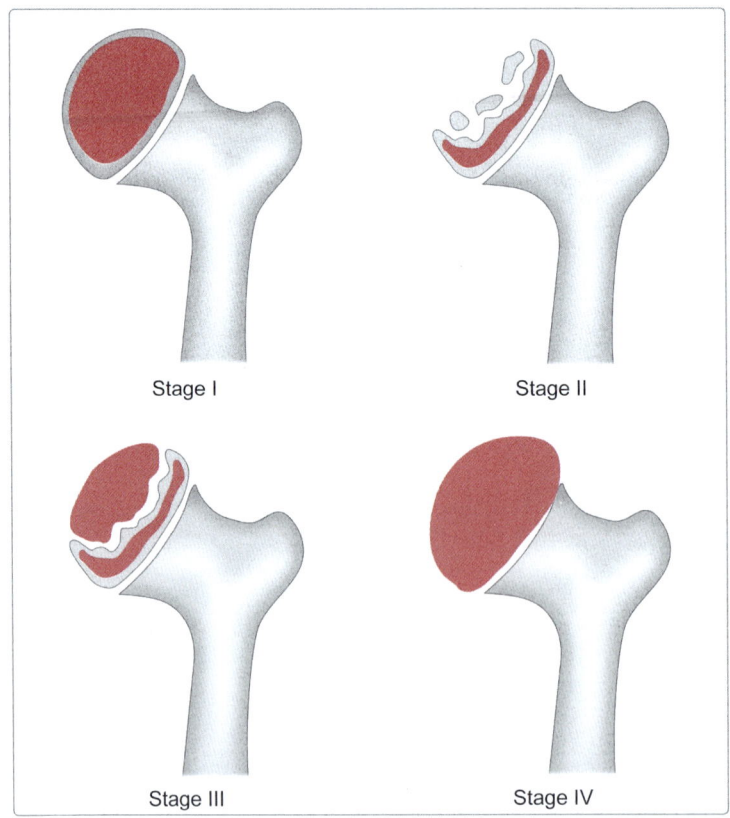

IV. *Healed:*
- *Stage IV:* Healing is complete and there is no radiologically identifiable avascular bone.

SLIPPED CAPITAL FEMORAL EPIPHYSIS

Grading of slipped capital femoral epiphysis (SCFE) can be made on both AP and true lateral projections.

On an AP radiograph: A line along the superior margin of the femoral neck (line of Klein) should intersect the lateral corner of the epiphysis. It is also known as **Trethowan's sign**.
- *Mild:* Lateral edge of epiphysis is within the lateral third of the metaphysis.
- *Moderate:* Middle third
- *Severe:* Medial third

On a true lateral radiograph: The angle (slip angle) which the epiphysis makes with the metaphysis is measured.
- *Normal:* 0°
- *Mild:* 0–30°
- *Moderate:* 30–60°
- *Severe:* >60°

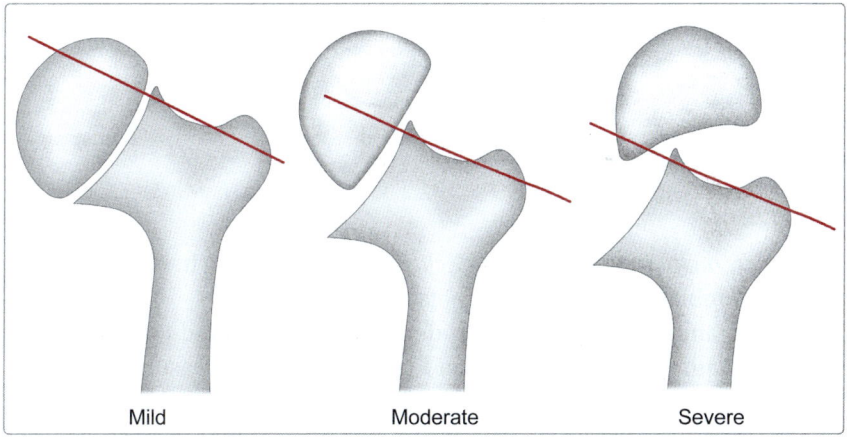

Mild   Moderate   Severe

DEVELOPMENTAL DYSPLASIA OF HIP

Crowe Classification

Type of classification for severity of adult developmental dysplasia of hip (DDH):
- *Grade 1:* Hips have less than 50% subluxation.
- *Grade 2:* Hips have between 50% and 75% subluxation.
- *Grade 3:* Hips have between 75% and 100% subluxation.
- *Grade 4:* Hips have more than 100% subluxation.

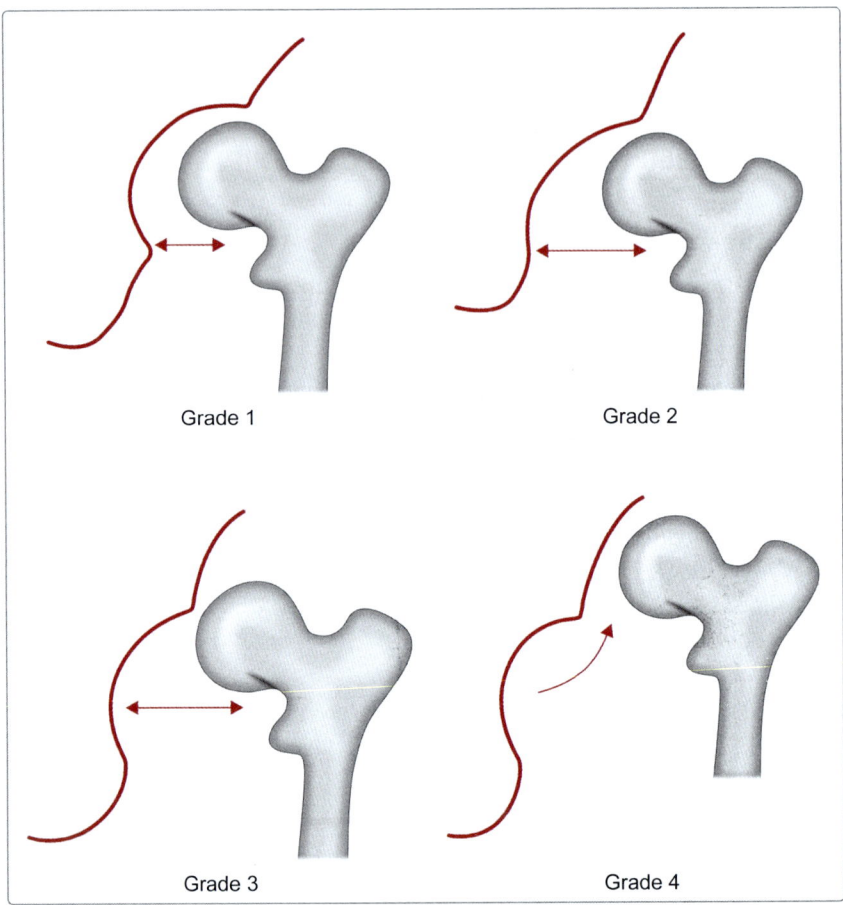

The Graf method for ultrasound classification system: It is for DDH in infants, combines both alpha and beta angles.

The infant remains in a lateral decubitus position and coronal images are taken with ultrasound probe and the two angles are measured.

The alpha angle refers to the angle between the acetabular roof and vertical cortex of the ilium. The beta angle is the angle formed between the vertical cortex of the ilium and the triangular labral fibrocartilage (echogenic triangle). In general, bigger the beta angle, greater the dysplasia. Therefore, **B**ig **B**eta **B**ad.

- *Type I:* Alpha angle > 60° (normal)
- *Type II:*
  - *Type IIa:* Alpha angle 50–59° (<3 months)
  - *Type IIb:* Alpha angle 50–59° (>3 months)
  - *Type IIc:*
    - Alpha angle 43–49°
    - Beta angle 70–77°

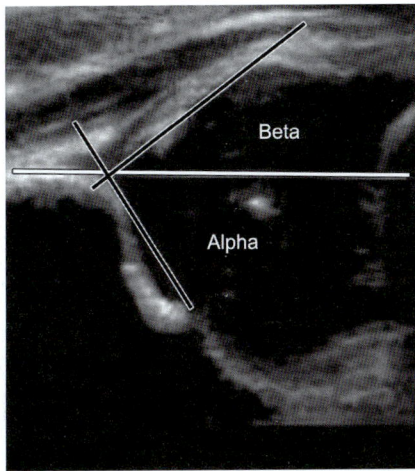

Ultrasound of the affected hip in sagittal plane showing alpha and beta angles.

- *Type IId:*
    - Alpha angle 43–49°
    - Beta angle > 77°
- *Type III:*
    - Alpha angle < 43°
    - Type IIIa and IIIb distinguished on the grounds of structural alteration of the cartilaginous roof
- *Type IV:*
    - Alpha angle < 43°
    - Dislocated with labrum interposed between the femoral head and acetabulum
    - Inverted labrum

AVASCULAR NECROSIS

The Ficat and Arlet Classification
- *Stage 0:* No clinical features with no findings in X-ray and MRI scan.
- *Stage I:* Pain typically in the groin region with plain radiograph showing normal or minor osteopenia, MRI shows bone edema and increased uptake in bone scan.
- *Stage IIa:* Pain and stiffness present.
    - X-ray shows subchondral cysts, without any subchondral lucency.
    - MRI: Geographic defect
    - Bone scan: Increased uptake
- *Stage IIb:* Pain and stiffness. Pain may be radiating to knee associated with limp.
    - X-ray crescent sign (subchondral lucency) and eventual cortical collapse
    - MRI: Same as plain radiograph

- *Stage III:* Broken contour of femoral head, bone sequestrum, joint space normal
- *Stage IV:* Pain associated with limp
  - X-ray and MRI scan shows end-stage with evidence of secondary degenerative changes in femur and acetabulum with joint space narrowing.

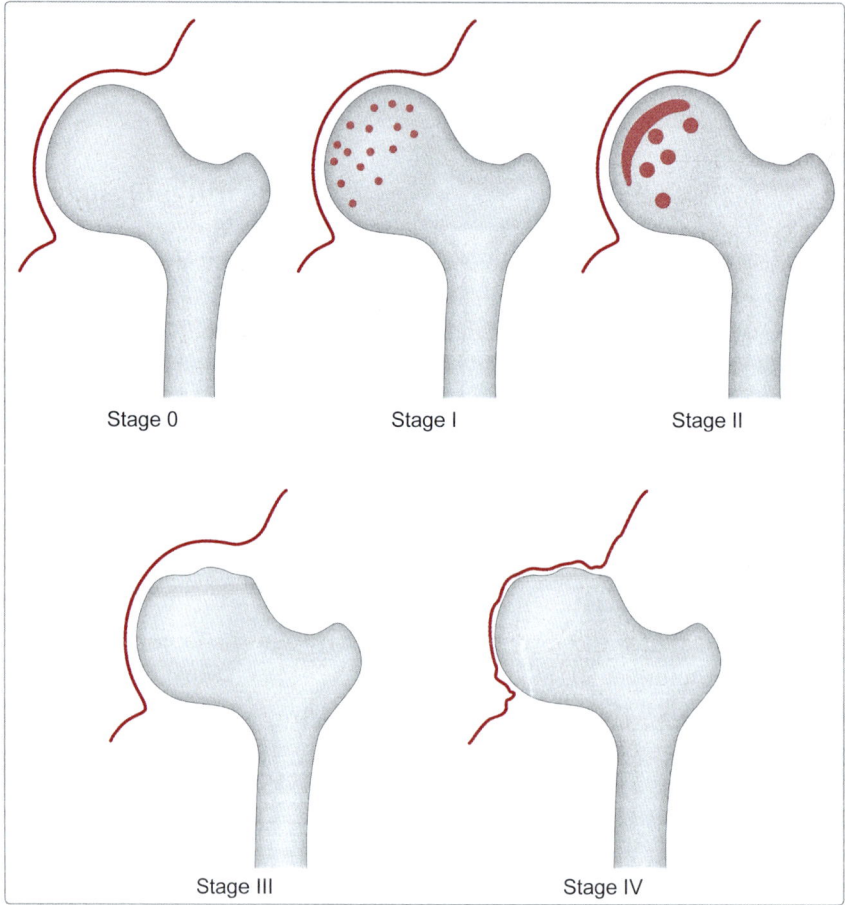

Steinberg Classification

- *Stage 0:* Normal or nondiagnostic radiographs, MRI and bone scan of at risk hip (often contralateral hip involved, or patient has risk factors and hip pain)
- *Stage I:* Normal radiograph, abnormal bone scan and/or MRI
- *Stage II:* Cystic and sclerotic radiographic changes
- *Stage III:* Subchondral lucency or crescent sign
- *Stage IV:* Flattening of femoral head, with depression graded into mild: <2 mm, moderate: 2–4 mm; severe: >4 mm

- *Stage V:* Joint space narrowing with or without acetabular involvement
- *Stage VI:* Advanced degenerative changes

Association Research Circulation Osseous (ARCO) Classification

Stage	Radiological findings
0	*Positive:* Histology; negative/normal: Radiograph/CT/MRI/scintigraphy
I	*Positive:* MRI and/or bone scintigraphy; negative/normal: radiograph/CT
II	*Radiograph:* Sclerotic, cystic or osteoporotic changes of femoral head
III	*Radiograph:* Subchondral fracture ("crescent sign")
IV	*Radiograph:* Flattening of femoral head++
V	*Radiograph:* Flattening of femoral head and osteoarthritic changes decreased joint space and acetabular changes++
VI	Complete joint destruction

FEMOROACETABULAR IMPINGEMENT

Ganz Subtypes

- *Cam impingement:* Due to abnormal shape of the femur head which is nonspherical.
- *Pincer impingement:* In this type, acetabular rim covers over the femur head. Shape of head normal.

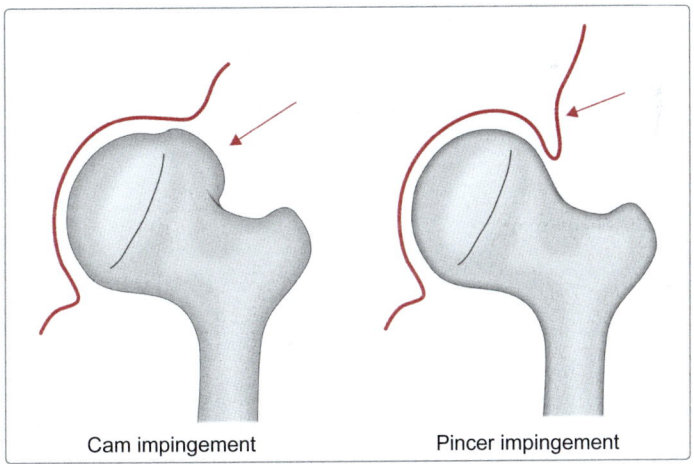

Cam impingement   Pincer impingement

OSTEOARTHRITIS

The Kellgren and Lawrence Classification

- *Grade 0:* No radiographic features of OA are present
- *Grade 1:* Doubtful joint space narrowing and possible osteophytic lipping

- *Grade 2:* Definite osteophytes and possible joint space narrowing on AP weight-bearing radiograph
- *Grade 3:* Multiple osteophytes, definite joint space narrowing, sclerosis, possible bony deformity
- *Grade 4:* Large osteophytes, marked joint space narrowing, severe sclerosis and definite bony deformity

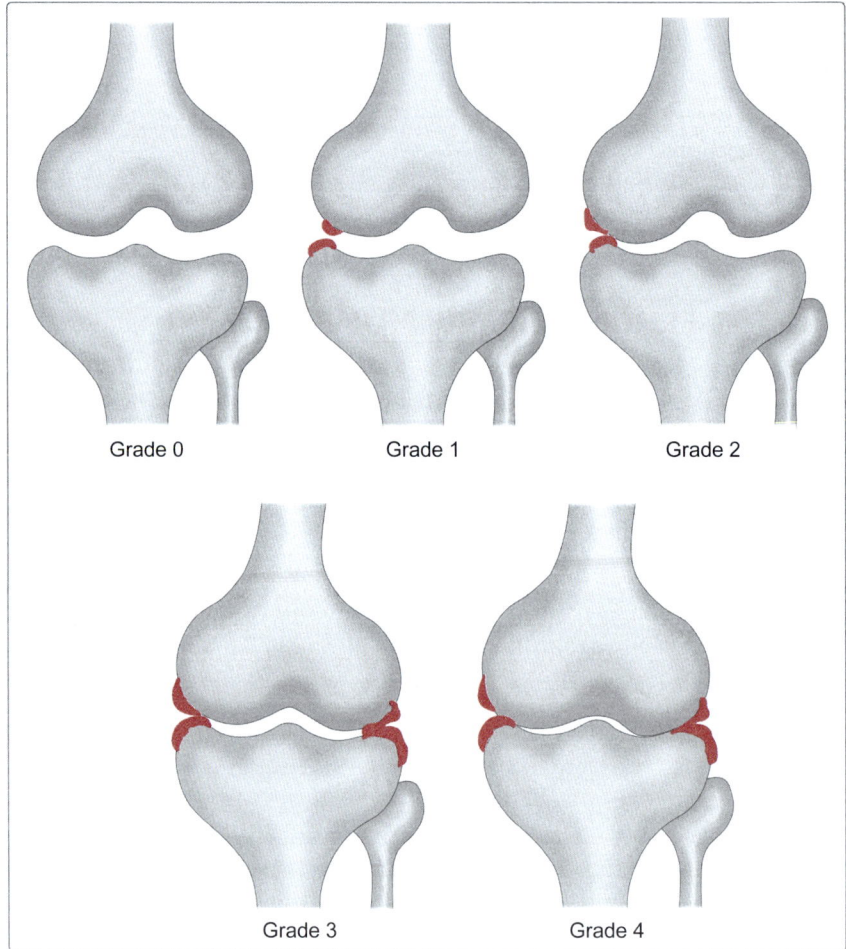

CHONDROMALACIA PATELLA

Outerbridge Classification

- *Grade 1:* Articular surfaces are soft
- *Grade 2:* Articular fissures and clefts with diameter < 1 cm
- *Grade 3:* Deep fissures with diameter extending > 1 cm
- *Grade 4:* Exposed subchondral bone

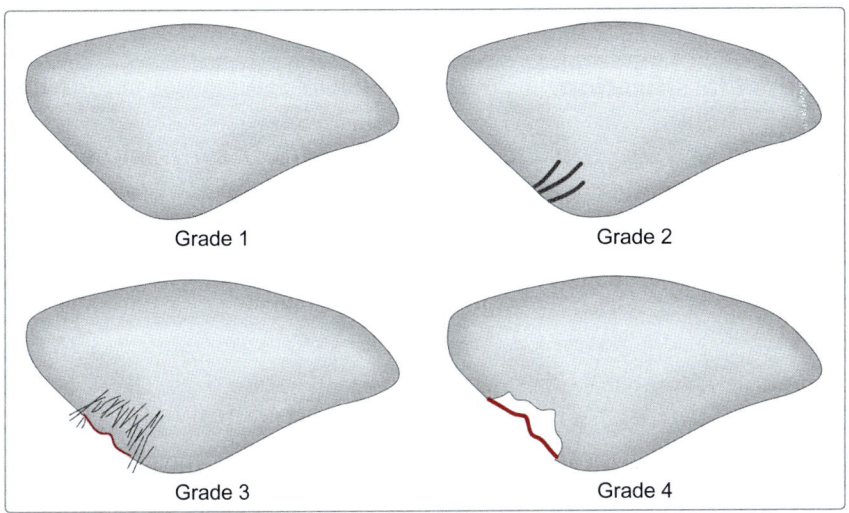

BIPARTITE PATELLA

Saupe Classification

- *Type 1:* Accessory center at the inferior pole
- *Type 2:* Occurs at the lateral border associated with nonunion of patella fracture
- *Type 3:* Occurs at the superolateral margin

ACCESSORY NAVICULAR

Kidner Classification

- *Type 1:* Round sesamoid within the tibialis posterior tendon
- *Type 2:* Synchondrosis within the body of navicular. Most common type (50%).
- *Type 3:* Fusion of accessory bone to the body of navicular.

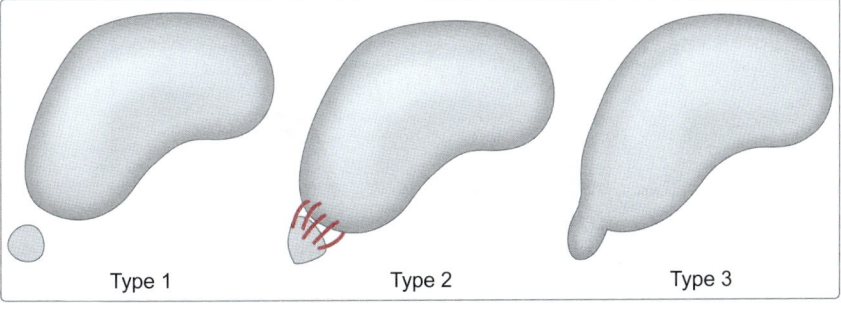

HALLUX VALGUS

Mann's Classification
- *Mild:* <25°
- *Moderate:* >25°, <40°
- *Severe:* >40°

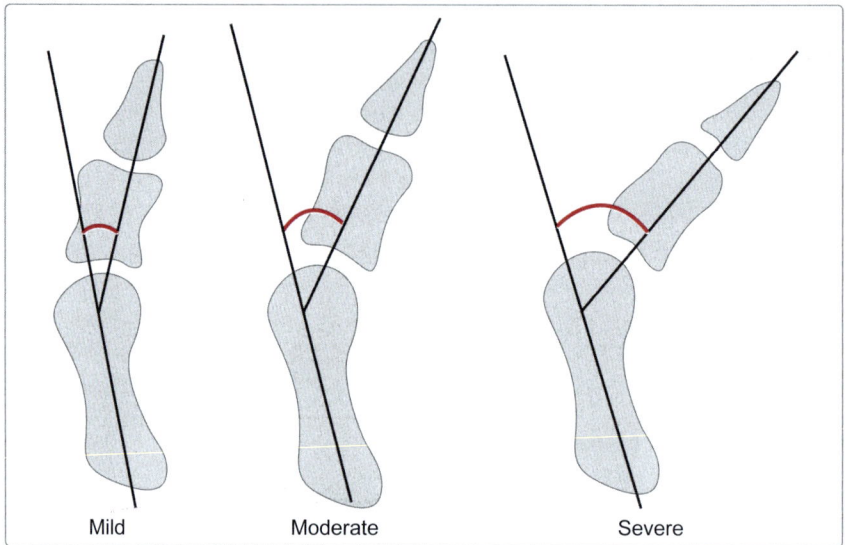

OSTEOCHONDRITIS DISSECANS OF TALUS

Berndt and Harty Classification
- *Stage I:* Subchondral bone compression (marrow edema)
- *Stage II:*
  - *Stage IIa:* Subchondral cyst
  - *Stage IIb:* Incomplete separation of fragment

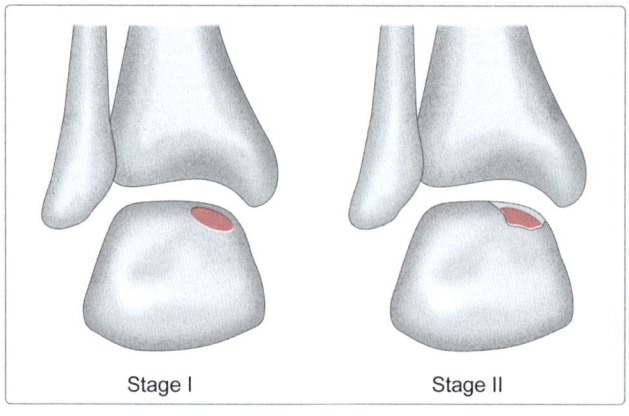

- *Stage III:* Complete separation but no displacement
- *Stage IV:* Displaced fragment

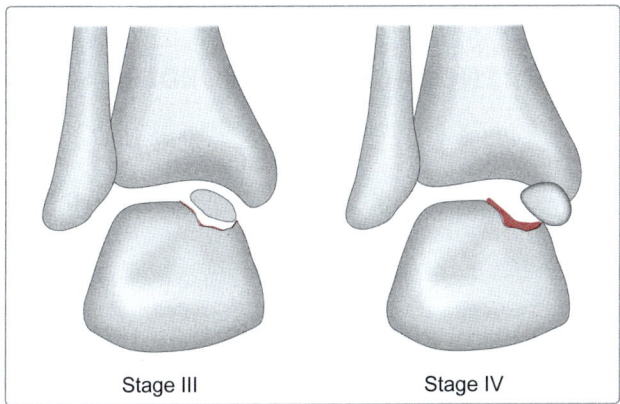

DIABETIC FOOT

Wagner Classification

It assesses ulcer depth and the presence of osteomyelitis or gangrene.
- *Grade 0:* Intact skin
- *Grade 1:* Superficial ulcer of skin or subcutaneous tissue
- *Grade 2:* Ulcers extend into tendon, bone, or capsule
- *Grade 3:* Deep ulcer with osteomyelitis, or abscess
- *Grade 4:* Partial foot gangrene
- *Grade 5:* Whole foot gangrene

Ganga Diabetic Foot Classification

- *Class 1:* Foot at risk
- *Class 2:* Superficial ulcers without infection
- *Class 3:* Crippled foot
- *Class 4:* Critical foot

CHARCOT'S ARTHROPATHY

Eichenholtz Classification

- *Stage 0:* Clinically, there is joint edema, but radiographs are negative. Note that a bone scan may be positive before a radiograph is, making it a sensitive but not very specific modality.
- *Stage 1:* Osseous fragmentation with joint dislocation seen on radiograph ("acute Charcot").

- *Stage 2:* Decreased local edema, with coalescence of fragments and absorption of fine bone debris.
- *Stage 3:* No local edema, with consolidation and remodeling (albeit deformed) of fracture fragments. The foot is now stable.

TENDOACHILLES DISORDERS

- *Insertional tendinitis:* Retrocalcaneal bursitis
- *Noninsertional tendinitis:*
  - Peritendinitis
  - Peritendinitis with tendinosis
  - Tendinosis

TIBIALIS POSTERIOR INSUFFICIENCY

Tendo Achilles Chronic Injury Classification

Myerson Algorithm

- *Type 1:* 1–2 cm tear (Direct repair)
- *Type 2:* 2–5 cm tear (V-Y advancement/Tendon transfer)
- *Type 3:* >5 cm tear (Tendon transfer)

Kuwada Algorithm

- *Type 1:* Partial tears (Conservative management)
- *Type 2:* Complete tears with <3 cm gap (Direct repair)
- *Type 3:* 3–6 cm gap (tendon graft)
- *Type 4:* >6 cm gap (Gastrocnemius recession with tendon graft)

Johnson and Strom Classification

- *Stage 1:* It is characterized by swelling, pain, inflammation, and effusion of the tendon sheath. No deformity of the foot. Able to invert the foot.
- *Stage 2:* It is characterized by loss of function of tibialis posterior and inability to perform single-toe raise.
- *Stage 3:* Loss of function with fixed hindfoot deformity. Degenerative changes present.
- *Stage 4:* Degenerative changes with valgus positioning of the ankle.

Spinal Disorders

LUMBAR CANAL STENOSIS

Anatomic Classification

- *Central stenosis:* It is caused by ligamentum hypertrophy directly under the lamina posteriorly and the bulging disk anteriorly. Cross sectional area is <100 mm^2.
- *Lateral recess stenosis:* It is caused by facet joint arthropathy and osteophyte formation.
- *Foraminal stenosis:* It occurs between the medial and lateral border of the pedicle due to loss of disk height or degenerative angulation.
- *Extraforaminal stenosis:* It is caused by far lateral disk herniations.

Classification Based on MRI

- *Type I:* Normal canal
- *Type IIa:* Tapering of the spinal canal at TL junction peaking at L5S1
- *Type IIb:* Hourglass constriction peaking at TL junction
- *Type III:* Global stenosis at all lumbar levels

SPONDYLOLISTHESIS

Meyerding's Classification

- *Grade I* spondylolisthesis is 1-25% slippage.
- *Grade II* is up to 50% slippage.
- *Grade III* is up to 75% slippage.
- *Grade IV* is 76-100% slippage.
- *Grade V:* More than 100% slippage, it is known as spondyloptosis.

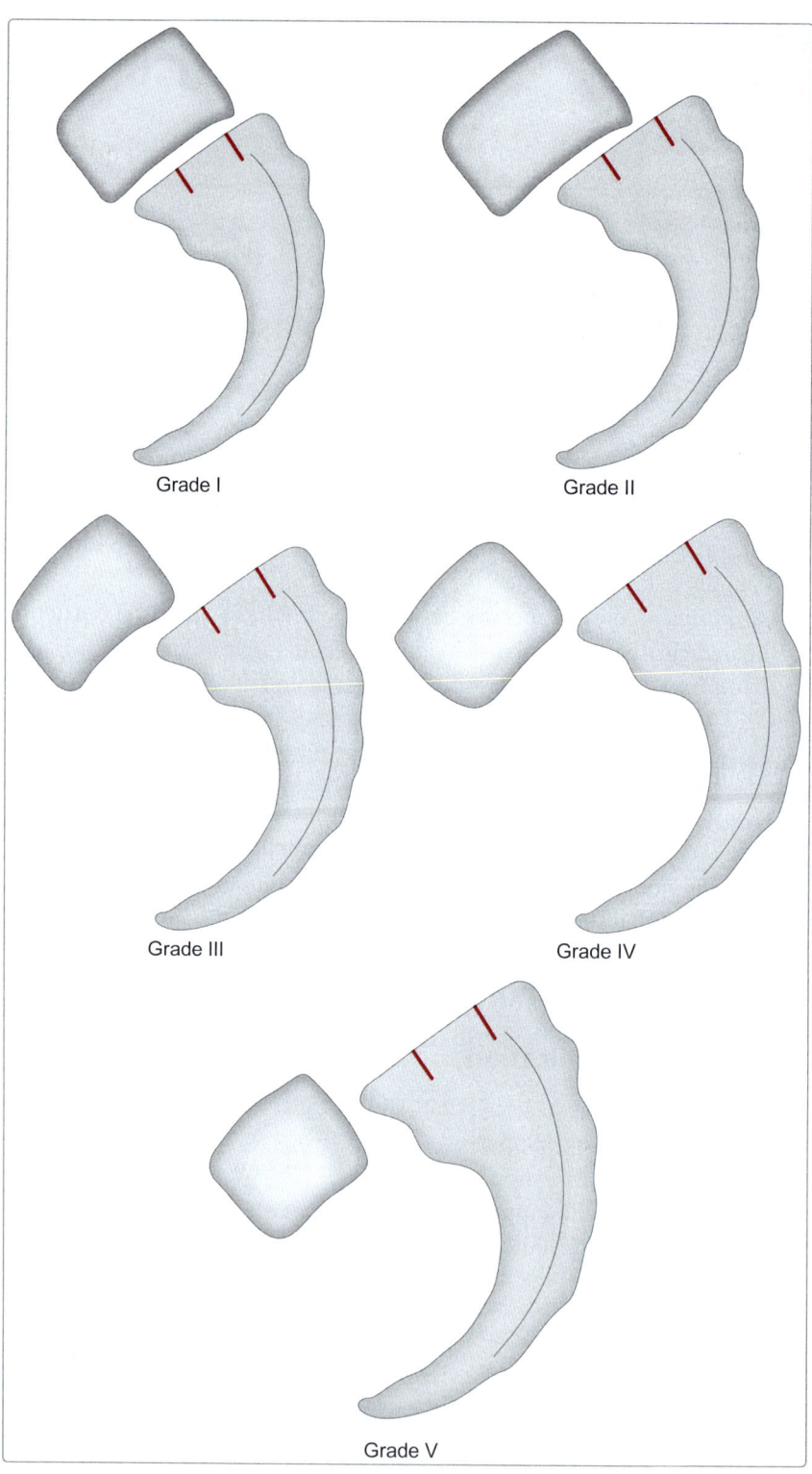

Grade I

Grade II

Grade III

Grade IV

Grade V

Wiltse-Newman Classification

- *Type I: Dysplastic spondylolisthesis* due to congenital defect in pars
- *Type II: Isthmic spondylolisthesis,* is caused by pars interarticularis fractures. Subclasses of isthmic spondylolisthesis are subtype A (stress fractures of the pars), subtype B (elongation of the pars without overt fracture), subtype C (acute fracture of the pars).
- *Type III: Degenerative spondylolisthesis,* is secondary to articular degeneration.
- *Type IV: Traumatic spondylolisthesis,* is caused by fracture or dislocation of the lumbar spine, not involving the pars.
- *Type V: Pathologic spondylolisthesis,* is caused by generalized or local bone disease.

KYPHOSIS

- Postural kyphosis
- Scheuermann's kyphosis
  - Thoracic
  - Thoracolumbar
  - Lumbar
- Congenital kyphosis
  - Failure of formation
  - Failure of segmentation
  - Combined
- Nutritional kyphosis
- Gibbus deformity is a form of structural kyphosis, often sequelae to tuberculosis.
- Post-traumatic kyphosis

INTERVERTEBRAL DISK PROLAPSE

- *Disk degeneration:* Loss of fluid in nucleus pulposus
- *Disk protrusion:* Disk bulges, but no rupture
- *Disk prolapse:* Nucleus pulposus is forced into the outermost layer of annulus fibrosus, no rupture.
- *Disk extrusion:* A small rupture occurs that allow fluid to enter epidural space.
- *Disk sequestration:* Free disk fragment lying outside

CHAPTER 8

Congenital Anomalies

WINGING OF SCAPULA

- Primary
  - *Neurogenic origin:*
    - Spinal accessory nerve
    - Long thoracic nerve
    - Dorsal scapular nerve
  - *Osseous origin:*
    - Osteochondromas
    - Fracture malunion
  - *Soft-tissue origin:*
    - Contractural winging
    - Muscular avulsion
    - Scapulothoracic bursitis
- Secondary
- Voluntary

SPRENGEL'S SHOULDER

Cavendish Classification

- *Grade I:*
  - Very mild deformity is observed.
  - When covered with clothes the deformity is almost invisible.
- *Grade II:*
  - The deformity is still mild but appears as a bump.
  - The superomedial portion of the high scapula is convex, forming a bump.
- *Grade III:* Moderate deformity with 2–5 cm of visible elevation of the affected shoulder
- *Grade IV:* Severe deformity with >5 cm elevation of the affected shoulder, accompanied by neck webbing

TORTICOLLIS

- *Osseous:* Occipitocervical synostosis, basilar impression, odontoid anomalies
- *Nonosseous:* Congenital muscular torticollis
    - Cheng's clinical group:
        - Sternomastoid tumor group
        - Muscular group
        - Postural torticollis
- *Neurogenic:* Nervous system tumors, syringomyelia, Arnold-Chiari malformation

CONGENITAL RADIOULNAR SYNOSTOSIS

Cleary (Modified)

- *Type I:* Synostosis does not involve bone, associated with reduced radial head.
- *Type II:* Visible osseous synostosis, associated with normal reduced radial head.
- *Type III:* Visible osseous synostosis with a hypoplastic and posteriorly dislocated radial head.
- *Type IV:* Short osseous synostosis with an anteriorly dislocated mushroom shaped radial head.

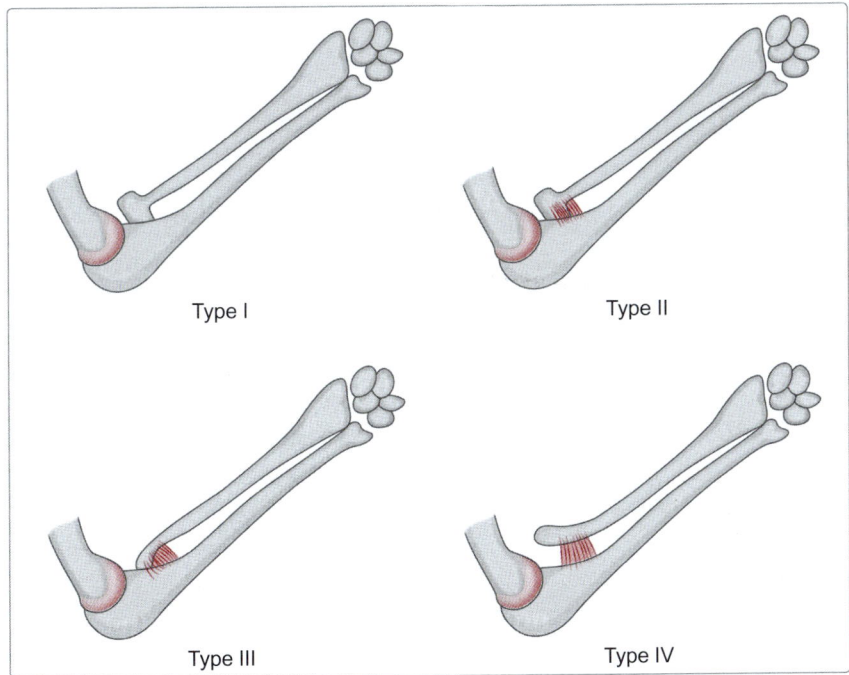

CONGENITAL HAND ANOMALIES

Swanson Classification

- *Failure of formation:* Radial club hand, ulnar club hand
- *Failure of differentiation:* Clinodactyly, syndactyly
- *Duplication:* Polydactyly
- *Overgrowth:* Macrodactyly
- *Undergrowth:* Thumb hypoplasia
- Congenital constriction band syndromes
- General skeletal abnormalities

Triphalangism

- *Type 1:* Rudimentary triphalangism
- *Type 2:* Triphalangism with a short triangular middle phalanx
- *Type 3:* Triphalangism with trapezoidal middle phalanx
- *Type 4:* Triphalangism with long rectangular middle phalanx
- *Type 5:* Hypoplastic triphalangeal thumb
- *Type 6:* Triphalangeal thumb associated with polydactyly

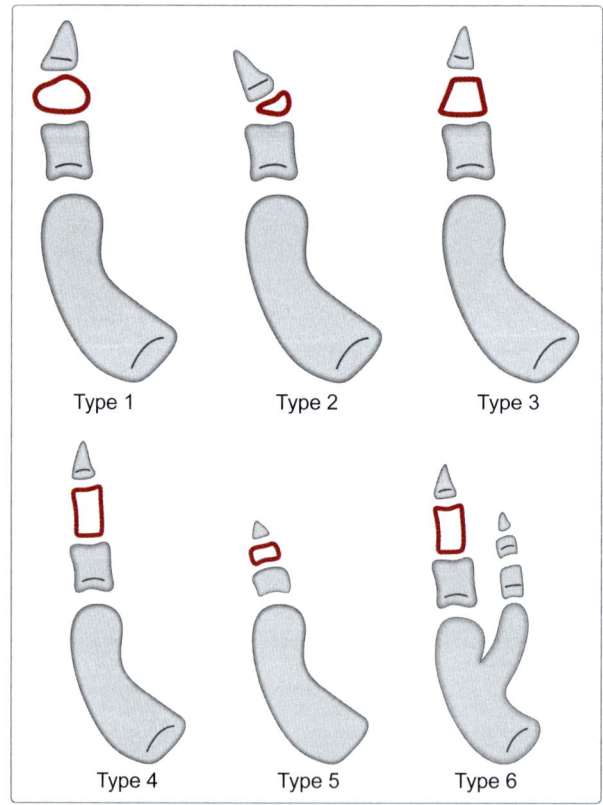

RADIAL CLUB HAND

Heikel Classification

- *Type 1—Short distal radius:* The distal radial physis is present but is delayed in appearance, the proximal radial physis is normal, ulna is bowed.
- *Type 2—Hypoplastic radius:* Both distal and proximal radial physis are present but are delayed in appearance, which result in moderate shortening of the radius and thickening and bowing of the ulna.
- *Type 3—Partial absence of radius:* Deformity may be proximal, middle or distal. Absence of the distal third is the most common. The carpus radially deviates and the ulna is thickened and bowed.
- *Type 4—Total absence of the radius:*
  - Most common. Radial deviation of the carpus, palmar and proximal subluxation.
  - Carpus might show pseudoarticulation with the radial border of the distal ulna, and a shortened and bowed ulna.

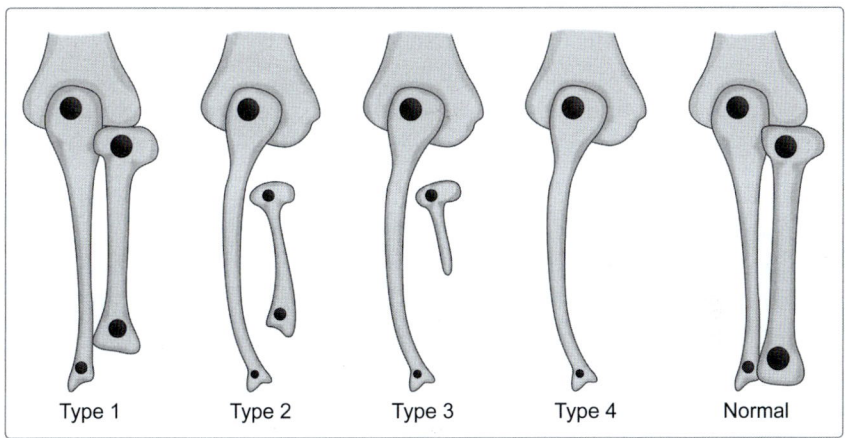

Note: Radial club hand may be associated with VACTERL. VACTERL is a nonrandom association of birth defects that affects multiple anatomical structures. The term VACTERL is an acronym with each letter representing the first letter of one of the more common findings seen in affected children: (V) = (costo-) vertebral abnormalities, (A) = anal atresia, (C) = cardiac defects, (TE) = tracheal-esophageal abnormalities, (R) = renal abnormalities, (L) = limb abnormalities, and (S) = single umbilical artery.

THUMB ANOMALY TYPES

- Duplication
- Triphalangia
- Flexed thumb
- Hypoplasia

HYPOPLASIA OF THUMB

Blauth Classification
- *Type 1:* Minimal shortening or narrowing
- *Type 2:* Narrow first web space, intrinsic muscle hypoplasia, MCP joint instability
- *Type 3A:* Narrow first web space, metacarpal hypoplasia with stable CMC joint
- *Type 3B:* Type 3A with unstable CMC joint
- *Type 4:* Rudimentary phalanges
- *Type 5:* Aplastic thumb

SYNDACTYLY

Temtamy and McKusick are described following five types:
- *Type 1:* Zygodactyly (syndactyly between 3rd and 4th fingers)
- *Type 2:* Synpolydactyly (syndactyly between 3rd and 4th fingers associated with a partial and a complete reduplication of the 3rd or 4th fingers in the webspace)
- *Type 3:* Ring and little fingers syndactyly
- *Type 4:* Complete syndactyly of all fingers
- *Type 5:* Syndactyly associated with metacarpal and metatarsal synostosis.

APERT SYNDROME

Blauth and Schneider gave a functional classification:
- *Type 1:* Only the central digits are fused. The thumb is well defined from the rest of the digital complex, but its range of movement is restricted by insufficient depth and width of webspace. The little finger too, appears well segmented from the outside and is tethered to its neighbor only by a partial soft tissue bridge.
- *Type 2:* (Obstetric hand) the little finger forms part of the total (nonosseous) syndactylous mass.

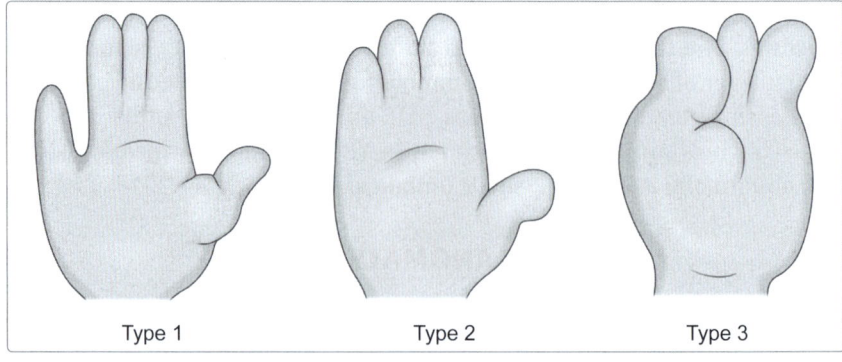

- *Type 3:* (Spoon hand) constitutes the most severe form, with complete syndactyly involving the thumb and all of the fingers. The fingertips are roughly level, with palmar cupping and fused. They are covered by a confluent nail, which often shows a roof-like deformity.

RING CONSTRICTION SYNDROME

- *Type 1:* Simple constriction rings
- *Type 2:* Constriction rings associated with deformity of distal part with or without lymphedema or atrophy (hypoplasia)
- *Type 3:* Constriction ring associated with soft tissue fusions of distal parts (acrosyndactyly)
- *Type 4:* Intrauterine amputations (partial aplasia)

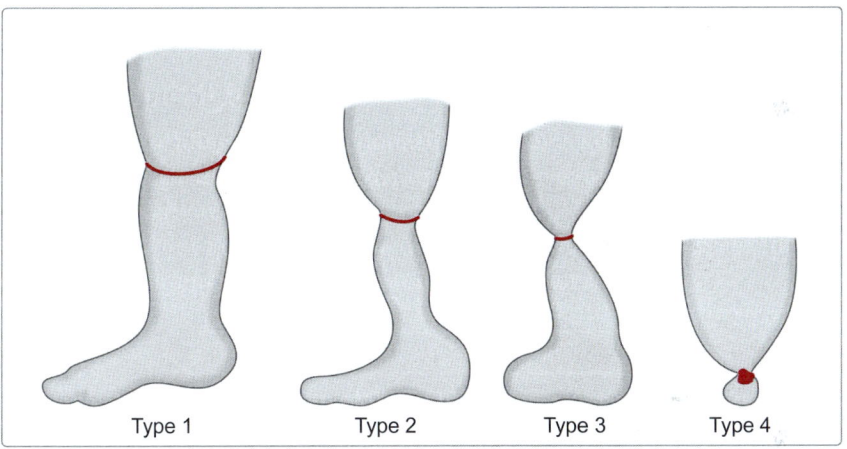

ULNAR CLUB HAND

Swanson Classification

- *Type 1:* Hypoplasia or partial defect of the ulna
- *Type 2:* Total defect of ulna
- *Type 3:* Total or partial defect of the ulna with humeroradial synostosis
- *Type 4:* Total or partial defect of the ulna associated with congenital amputation of the wrist.

MADELUNG DEFORMITY

Vender and Watson Classification

- Post-traumatic
- Genetic
- Dysplastic
- Idiopathic

PROXIMAL FEMORAL FOCAL DEFICIENCY

Aitken's Classification

- *Class A:* Normal acetabulum and femur head with shortening of the femur and absence of the femur neck on early X-rays. It may be associated with pseudarthrosis of the neck. Severe coxa vara with shortening of the limb.
- *Class B:* There is no bony connection between the proximal femur and head. Pseudarthrosis is present.
- *Class C:* There is dysplastic acetabulum, absent femur head and short femur. A small separate ossific tuft at the proximal femur.
- *Class D:* The acetabulum, femur head and the proximal femur are totally absent. There is no ossified tuft capping the proximal femur.

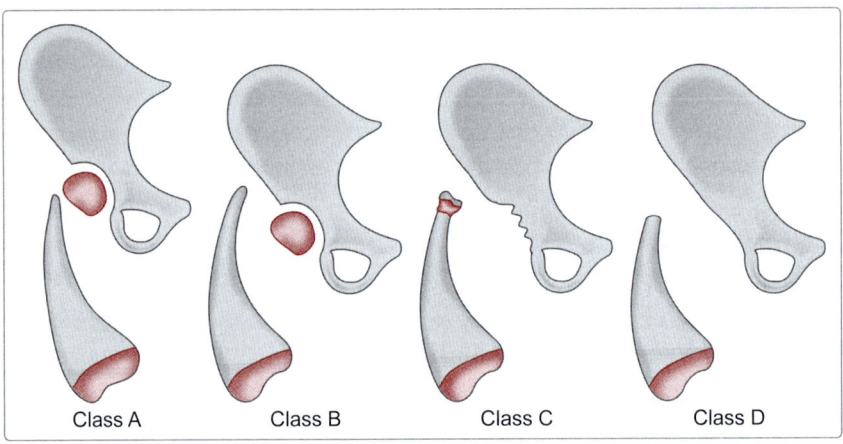

Kalamchi Classification

- *Group 1:* Short femur and intact hip joint
- *Group 2:* Short femur and coxa vara of the hip
- *Group 3:* Short femur but well developed acetabulum and femur head
- *Group 4:* Absent hip joint and dysplastic femoral segment
- *Group 5:* Total absence of femur

BLOUNT'S DISEASE/CONGENITAL TIBIA VARA

Langenskiold Classification

- *Stage I:* Irregularity of entire metaphysis. Medial metaphyseal beaking
- *Stage II:* Sharp anteromedial depression. There is a propensity for healing at this stage.
- *Stage III:* Deepening of the depression makes a step.
- *Stage IV:* Developed step is filled in by the epiphysis. Growth plate is irreversibly damaged at this stage.

- *Stage V:* A triangular fragment separates.
- *Stage VI:* Medial growth plate ossification. Growth continues in the normal lateral part.

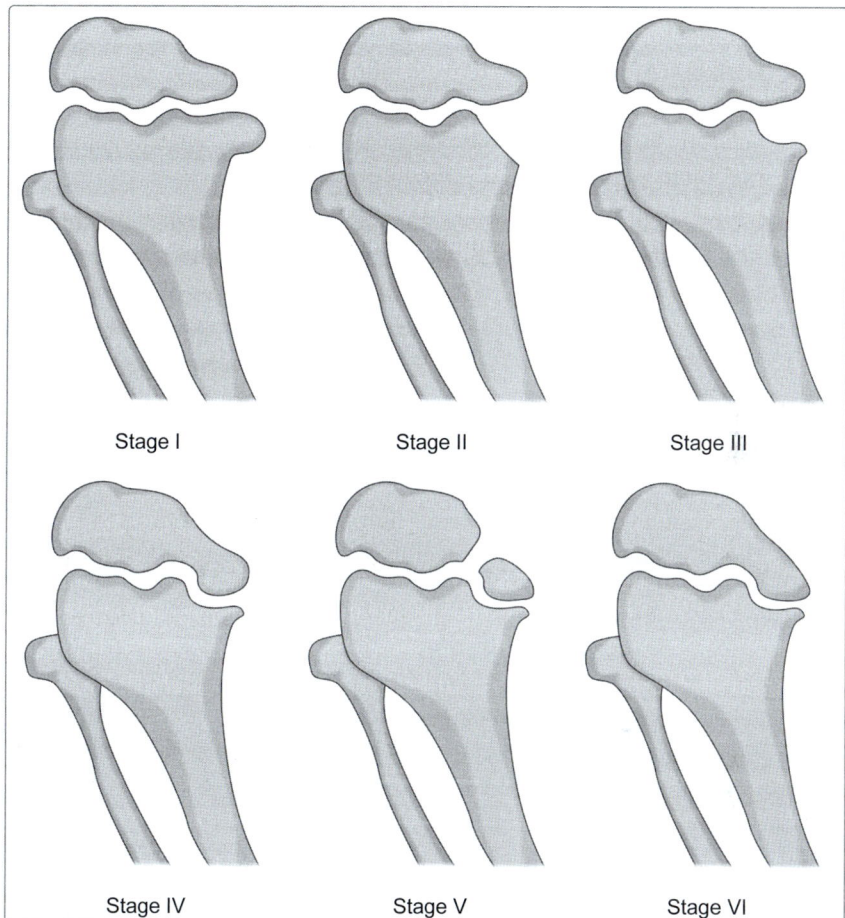

CONGENITAL PSEUDARTHROSIS OF TIBIA

Boyd Classification

It has six types and provides prognostic value:
- *Type I:* Anterior bowing associated with other congenital malformations.
- *Type II:*
  - Anterior bowing with an hourglass appearance to the tibia.
  - Fracture usually occurs before the age of 2 years.
  - The ends of the bone are thin, rounded, and sclerotic with obliteration of the intramedullary canal.

- Often associated with NF1.
- Poor prognosis with frequent recurrence.
  ○ *Type III:*
    - Pseudarthrosis developing from an intraosseous cyst.
    - Anterior bowing can precede or follow the development of the fracture.
    - High rate of union and rare recurrence.
  ○ *Type IV:*
    - Sclerotic bone with no pathological bowing.
    - Medullary canal is partially or completely obliterated.
    - Fatigue fracture may occur and progress to pseudarthrosis.
    - Good prognosis with treatment before fatigue fracture.
  ○ *Type V:*
    - Dysplastic appearance to the fibula.
    - Pseudarthrosis can be located on either of the two bones of the tibial segment.
    - The prognosis is good if the lesion is located only on the fibula, extension to the tibia has a prognosis similar to type II.
  ○ *Type VI:*
    - Associated with an intraosseous fibroma or a schwannoma.
    - Prognosis depends on how aggressive the intraosseous lesion is.

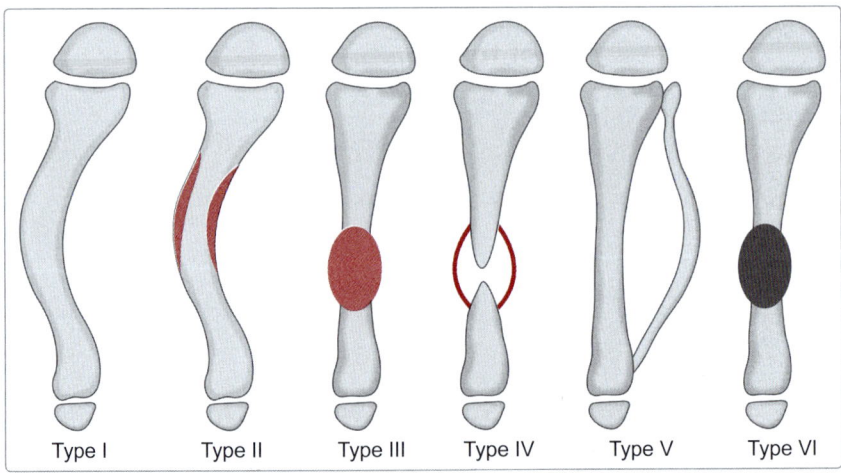

Crawford Classification
  ○ *Type 1:* Anterolateral bowing of tibia
  ○ *Type 2:*
    - Anterolateral bowing
    - Increased cortical thickness

- Narrow medullary canal
- Tubular defect
○ *Type 3:* Cystic lesion
○ *Type 4:* Frank pseudarthrosis

CONGENITAL TALIPES EQUINOVARUS

Pirani Scoring

Each component may score 0, 0.5 or 1 (if the sign is severely abnormal it scores 1, if it is partially abnormal it scores 0.5, if it is normal it scores 0).
○ *Hindfoot contracture score (HFCS):*
- Posterior crease
- Empty heel
- Rigid equinus
○ *Midfoot contracture score (MFCS):*
- Medial crease
- Curvature of lateral border
- Position of head of talus

Note: Feel of emptiness of heel can be assessed as follows: Score 1 is as if pressing your lip, score 0.5 is as if pressing your cartilaginous part of nose and score 0 is as if pressing your hard bony forehead.

Dimeglio Scoring

The Dimeglio scoring system includes the visual estimation of the equinus, hindfoot varus, midfoot rotation, and forefoot adduction without forcing the foot.

Each feature is given 0–4 points according to reducibility on the relative plane:
○ 90–45° = 4
○ 45–20° = 3
○ 20–0° = 2
○ 0–20° = 1
○ <20° = 0

Pejorative elements (posterior crease, medial crease, cavus, and muscular abnormality) were each scored as 1 if present and 0 if absent.

The total scale ranged from 0 to 20, with a score of 0 for a normal foot, ≤5 a benign deformity foot, 6–10 a moderate deformity foot, 11–15 a severe deformity foot and 16–20 a very severe deformity foot.

CONGENITAL VERTICAL TALUS

Hamanishi Classification

- *Type 1:* Vertical talus associated with spinal abnormalities
- *Type 2:* Vertical talus associated with neuromuscular disorders
- *Type 3:* Congenital vertical talus (CVT) associated with malformation syndromes
- *Type 4:* CVT associated with chromosomal anomalies
- *Type 5:*
  - *Type 5a:* Resulting from intrauterine disorder
  - *Type 5b:* With digitotalar dysmorphism
  - *Type 5c:* With vertical talus in a close relative
  - *Type 5d:* Not associated with any other skeletal anomaly or genetic component

TIBIA HEMIMELIA

Jones, Barnes, Lloyd-Roberts Classification

- *Type 1A:* There is complete absence of tibia and hypoplastic distal femur epiphysis.
- *Type 1B:* Distal femur epiphysis appears normal in size and shape. Proximal tibial anlage present.
- *Type 2:* Proximal tibia of varying size present with fibular head dislocated proximally.
- *Type 3:* Proximal tibia is absent. Distal tibia is present with mature tibial metaphysis: knee is unstable. This is the least common type.
- *Type 4:* There is shortened tibia with proximal migration of the fibula with distal tibiofibular diastasis.

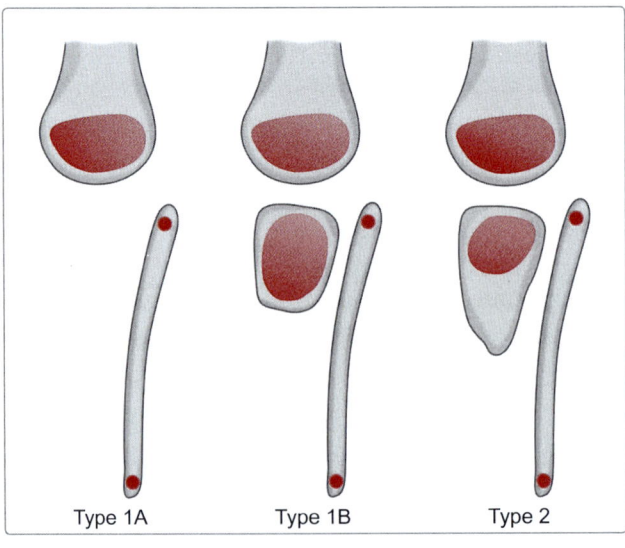

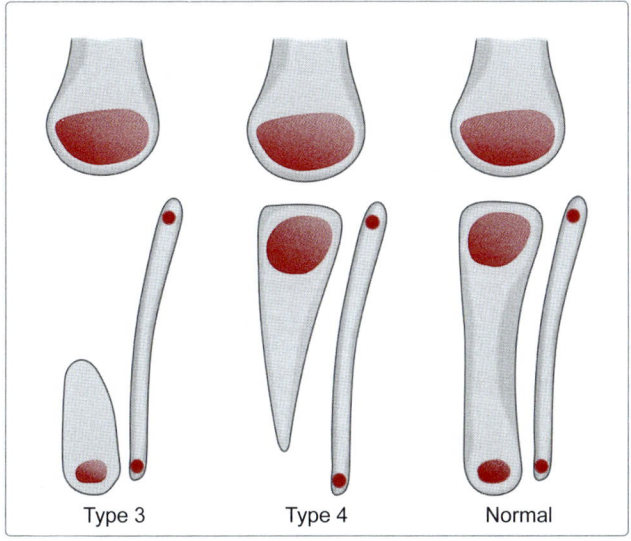

FIBULAR HEMIMELIA

Achterman and Kalamchi Classification

- *Type 1:* Hypoplasia of the fibula
  - *Type 1A:* Proximal fibula epiphysis is distal to the proximal tibial epiphysis and the distal fibular epiphysis is proximal to the talar dome.
  - *Type 1B:* 30–50% of the length of the fibula is missing and no distal support for the ankle.
- *Type 2:* Complete absence of the fibula. Angulation of the tibia is common in this type.

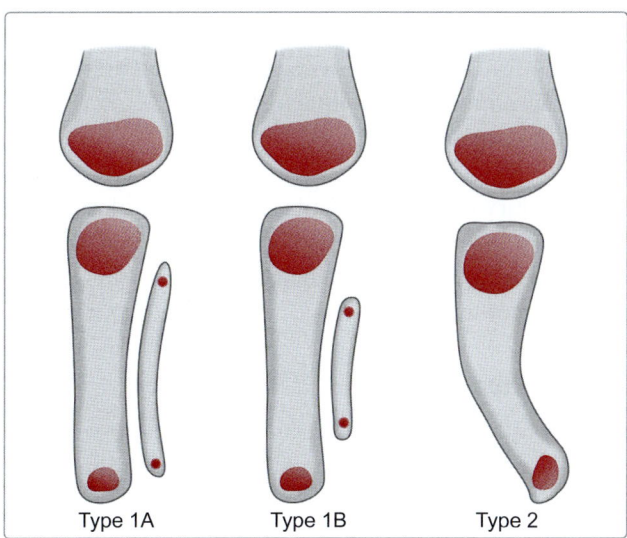

CHAPTER 9

Miscellaneous Conditions

OPEN FRACTURE

Gustilo-Anderson Classification

- *Type I:*
  - Wound ≤1 cm
  - Minimal contamination or muscle damage
  - Simple fracture
- *Type II:*
  - Wound 1-10 cm
  - Moderate soft tissue injury
  - Moderate comminution of fracture
  - Moderate contamination
- *Type IIIA:*
  - Wound usually >10 cm
  - High energy trauma, severe comminution/segmental fracture
  - Extensive soft-tissue damage, minimal periosteal stripping
  - Extensively contaminated
  - Adequate tissue for flap coverage
  - Farm injuries are automatically at least Gustilo IIIA
- *Type IIIB:*
  - Extensive periosteal stripping
  - Wound requires soft tissue coverage (rotational or free flap)
  - Severe comminution/segmental fracture
  - Extensively contaminated
- *Type IIIC:*
  - Vascular injury requiring vascular repair, regardless of degree of soft tissue injury
  - Severe comminution/segmental fracture
  - Extensively contaminated

Tscherne Classification

- *Grade I:*
  - Open fractures with a small puncture wound without skin contusion
  - Negligible bacterial contamination
  - Low-energy fracture pattern

- Grade II:
  - Open injuries with small skin and soft tissue contusions
  - Moderate contamination
  - Variable fracture patterns
- Grade III:
  - Open fractures with heavy contamination
  - Extensive soft tissue damage
  - Often, associated arterial or neural injuries
- Grade IV: Open fractures with incomplete or complete amputations

GAIT

- Stance:
  - Initial contact
  - Midstance
  - Preswing
  - Loading response
  - Terminal stance
- Swing:
  - Initial swing
  - Mid swing
  - Terminal swing

MANGLED EXTREMITY SEVERITY SCORE (MESS)

MANGLED EXTREMITY SEVERITY SCORE*	
Skeletal/Soft-tissue injury	**Points**
Low energy (stab; simple fracture; pistol GSW)	1
Medium energy (open or multiple fractures, dislocation)	2
High energy (high speed MVA or rifle GSW)	3
Very high energy (high speed trauma + gross contamination)	4
Limb ischemia	
Pulse reduced or absent but perfusion normal	1
Pulseless; paresthesias, diminished capillary refill	2
Cool, paralyzed, insensate, numb	3
Shock	
Systolic BP always >90 mm Hg	0
Hypotensive transiently	1
Persistent hypotension	2
Age (years)	
<30	0
30–50	1
50	2

*Score doubled for ischemia > 6 hours.
Interpretation: Score of >7 is predictive of amputation.
(GSW: gunshot wound; MVA: motor vehicle accident)

Miscellaneous Conditions

INJURY SEVERITY SCORE

Variables

Based on scores of nine anatomic regions:
- Head
- Face
- Neck
- Thorax
- Abdominal and pelvic contents
- Spine
- Upper extremity
- Lower extremity
- External

Calculation

Abbreviated Injury Scale (AIS) grades:
- 0—No injury
- 1—Minor
- 2—Moderate
- 3—Severe (not life-threatening)
- 4—Severe (life-threatening, survival probable)
- 5—Severe (critical, survival uncertain)
- 6—Maximal, possibly fatal

Injury severity score (ISS) = Sum of squares for the highest AIS grades in the three most severely injured ISS body regions:

$$ISS = A^2 + B^2 + C^2$$

where, A, B, and C are the AIS scores of the three most severely injured ISS body region.

Scores range from 1 to 75.

Single score of 6 on any AIS region results in automatic score of 75.

GANGA HOSPITAL SCORING SYSTEM

GANGA HOSPITAL SCORING SYSTEM	
Covering structures: Skin and fascia	**Score**
Wound with no skin loss and not over the fracture site	1
Wound with no skin loss and over the fracture site	2
Wound with skin loss and not over the fracture site	3
Wound with skin loss and over the fracture site	4
Wound with circumferential skin loss	5

Contd…

Contd...

Functional tissues: Musculotendinous and nerve units	Score
Partial injury to musculotendinous unit	1
Complete but repairable injury to musculotendinous units	2
Irreparable injury to musculotendinous units, partial loss of a compartment, or complete injury to posterior tibial nerve	3
Loss of one compartment of musculotendinous units	4
Loss of two or more compartments or subtotal amputation	5
Skeletal structures: Bone and joints	
Transverse or oblique fracture or butterfly fragment <50% circumference	1
Large butterfly fragment >50% circumference	2
Comminution or segmental fractures without bone loss	3
Bone loss <4 cm	4
Bone loss >4 cm	5

Comorbid conditions: Add two points for each condition present:
- Injury leading to debridement interval >12 hours
- Sewage or organic contamination or farmyard injuries
- Age > 65 years
- Drug-dependent diabetes mellitus or cardiorespiratory diseases leading to increased anesthetic risk
- Polytrauma involving chest or abdomen with injury severity score > 25 or fat embolism
- Hypotension with systolic blood pressure <90 mmHg at presentation
- Another major injury to the same limb or compartment syndrome

Interpretation:
- Injuries with a score equal to 14 or below are advised salvage.
- Injuries with score 17 and above usually end up in amputation.
- Injuries with score 15 and 16 fall into Gray zone where decision is made on patient to patient basis.

GLASGOW COMA SCALE (GCS)

Best Motor Response

- 6—Obeys command
- 5—Localizes pain
- 4—Normal withdrawal (flexion)
- 3—Abnormal withdrawal (flexion): Decorticate
- 2—Abnormal withdrawal (extension): Decerebrate
- 1—None (flaccid)

Best Verbal Response
- 5—Oriented
- 4—Confused conversation
- 3—Inappropriate words
- 2—Incomprehensible sounds
- 1—None

Eye Opening
- 4—Spontaneous
- 3—To speech
- 2—To pain
- 1—None

GCS-P: A modification of the GCS takes pupillary response into account. If one pupil is nonreactive to light, one point is subtracted from the total GCS score. If both pupils fail to constrict, two points are subtracted.

Brain Injury
- *Severe:* < 9
- *Moderate:* 9-12
- *Minor:* 13 and above

NONUNION

Weber Classification
- *Hypertrophic:*
  - Elephant foot
  - Horse hoof
  - Oligotrophic

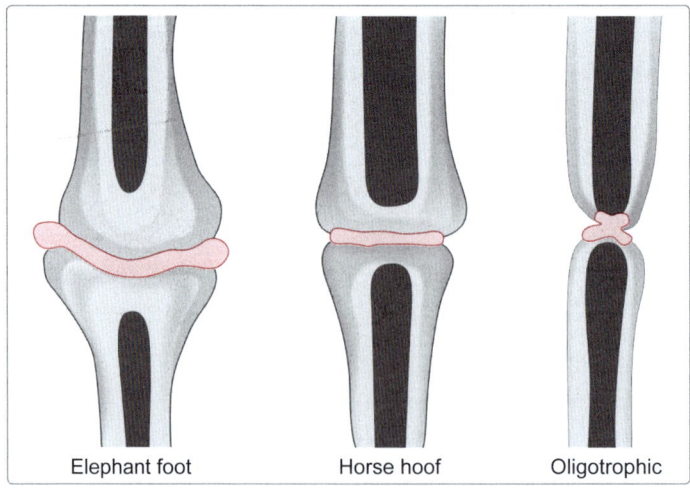

Elephant foot   Horse hoof   Oligotrophic

Miscellaneous Conditions

- *Atrophic:*
  - Torsion wedge
  - Comminuted
  - Defect
  - Atrophic

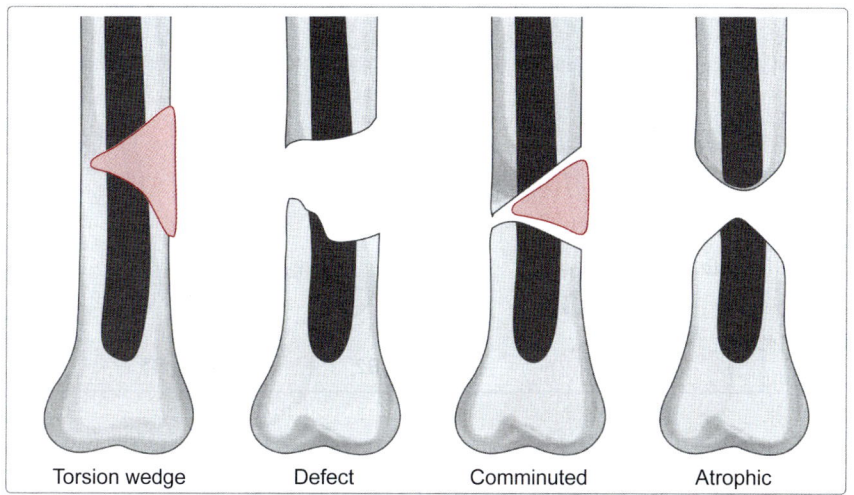

Paley Classification

- *Type A:* Bone loss less than 1 cm
  - *A1:* Nonunion with mobile deformity
  - *A2:* Stiff nonunion
    - *A2-1:* Stiff nonunion without deformity
    - *A2-2:* Stiff nonunion with deformity
- *Type B:* Bone loss more than 1 cm
  - *B1:* Bone defect only
  - *B2:* Shortening only
  - *B3:* Bone loss with shortening

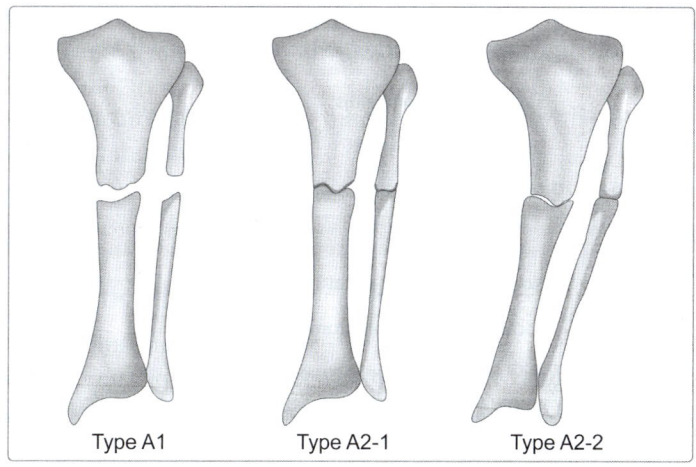

- *Type 2B:* Femur head deformity with growth arrest
- *Type 3:* Pseudoarthrosis of femur neck
- *Type 4A:* Complete destruction of the femur epiphysis with stable neck
- *Type 4B:* Complete destruction of the femur epiphysis with unstable neck segment
- *Type 5:* Complete destruction of head with dislocation

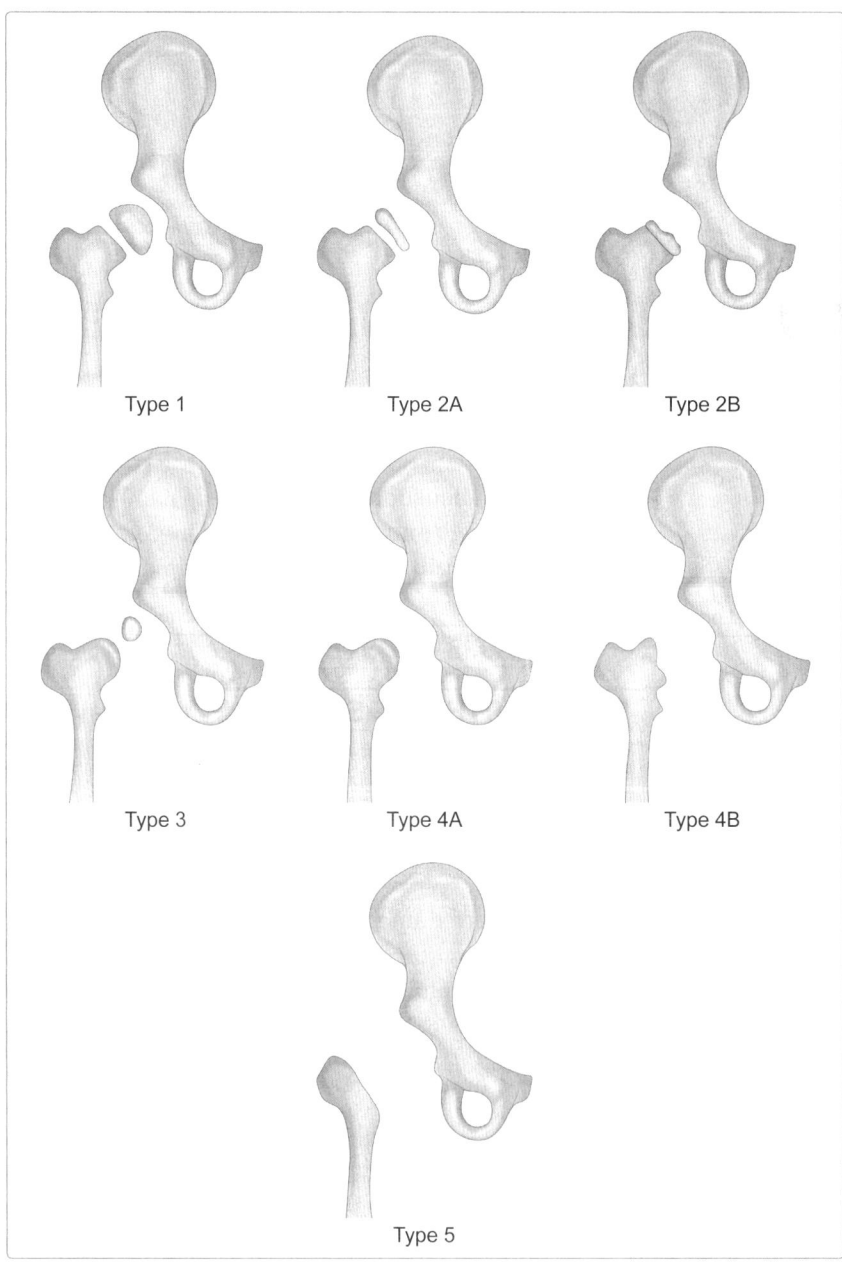

Choi's Classification

- *Type I:* Almost normal hip or mild coxa magna. It needs no reconstruction.
- *Type II:* Deformed epiphysis, physis, metaphysis may result in coxa breva or progressive coxa vara or coxa valgus. It needs surgical intervention to prevent subluxation.
- *Type III:* Malalignment of femoral neck, excessive anteversion or retroversion with pseudoarthrosis. It necessitates a realignment surgery for proximal femur or bone grafting for pseudoarthrosis.
- *Type IV:* Destruction of the head and neck of femur with the presence of remnant of medial base of neck. Complex clinical problems with limb length inequality need reconstructive surgery.

PIN TRACT SITE INFECTION

Checketts–Otterburn Grading

Grade	Appearance	Treatment
Minor infection		
1	Slight redness, little discharge	Improved pin site care
2	Redness of skin, discharge, pain and tenderness in the soft tissue	Improved pin site care, oral antibiotics
3	Grade 2 but not improved with antibiotics	Affected pin or pins resited and external fixation continued
Major infection		
4	Severe soft tissue infection involving several pins, sometimes with associated loosening of the pin	External fixation must be abandoned
5	Grade 4 but also involvement of the bone; also visible in radiographs	External fixation must be abandoned
6	The infection occurs after fixation removal. The pin track heals initially but will break down and discharge at intervals. Radiograph shows new bone formation and sometimes sequestrum	Curettage of the pin track

MALIGNANT TUMOR

Enneking Classification

Stage	Grade	Compartment	Metastasis
1A	Low	Intracompartmental	Nil
1B	Low	Extracompartmental	Nil
2A	High	Intracompartmental	Nil
2B	High	Extracompartmental	Nil
3	Low/High	Intracompartmental/Extracompartmental	Present

American Joint Committee on Cancer

AMERICAN JOINT COMMITTEE ON CANCER (AJCC) STAGING SYSTEM			
Stage	**Grade**	**Size**	**Metastases**
1A	Low	<8 cm	None
1B	Low	>8 cm	None
2A	High	<8 cm	None
2B	High	>8 cm	None
3	Any	Any	Skip
4A	Any	Any	Pulmonary
4B	Any	Any	Nonpulmonary

HEREDITARY MULTIPLE EXOSTOSES

Masada Classification

- *Type 1:* Primary exostoses in distal ulna with relatively short ulna
- *Type 2A:* Ulna shortening; radial head dislocated secondary to exostosis at the proximal radial metaphysis
- *Type 2B:* Radial head is dislocated without proximal radial head exostosis
- *Type 3:* Primary exostosis in the distal radial metaphysis with relatively short radius

GIANT CELL TUMOR

Campanacci Classification

- *Grade I (inactive):* Intraosseous lesion with intact cortex
- *Grade II (active):* Extensive intraosseous lesion with thin cortex
- *Grade III (aggressive):* Extraosseous lesion, fracture of cortex with soft tissue extension

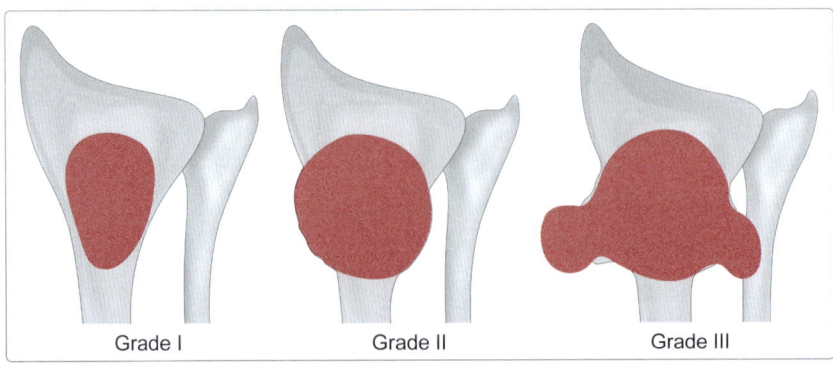

Grade I   Grade II   Grade III

PATTERN OF BONE DESTRUCTION

- *Type 1:* Geographic bone destruction
  - With sclerotic margin, e.g., chondroblastoma, fibrous dysplasia
  - Without sclerotic margin, e.g., giant cell tumor
  - With ill-defined margin, e.g., chondrosarcoma
- *Type 2:* Moth eaten appearance, e.g., Ewing's sarcoma, osteosarcoma
- *Type 3:* Permeative destruction, e.g., primary round cell tumors, osteomyelitis

PERIPROSTHETIC FRACTURE OF HIP

Vancouver Classification

Type	Fracture description
A	Fracture around the trochanteric region
B1	Fracture around the stem but well-fixed stem
B2	Fracture around the stem with loose stem; bone quality good
B3	Fracture around the stem with poor quality bone
C	Fracture below the prosthesis

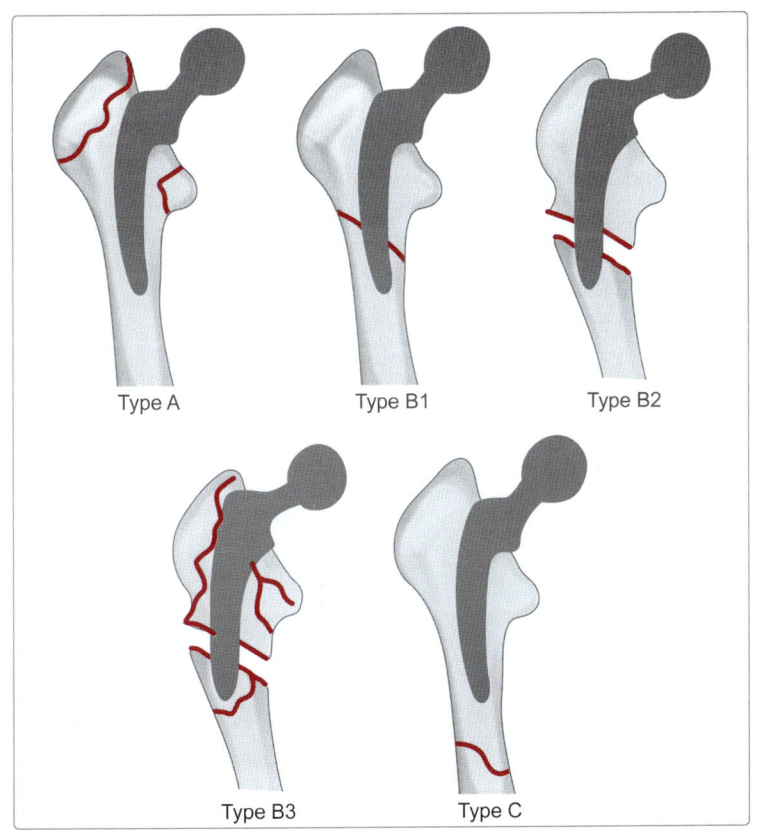

PERIPROSTHETIC FRACTURE AROUND KNEE

Femur

Lewis and Rorabeck Classification
- *Type I:* Undisplaced fracture, prosthesis stable
- *Type II:* Displaced fracture, prosthesis stable
- *Type III:* Unstable prosthesis with or without fracture displacement

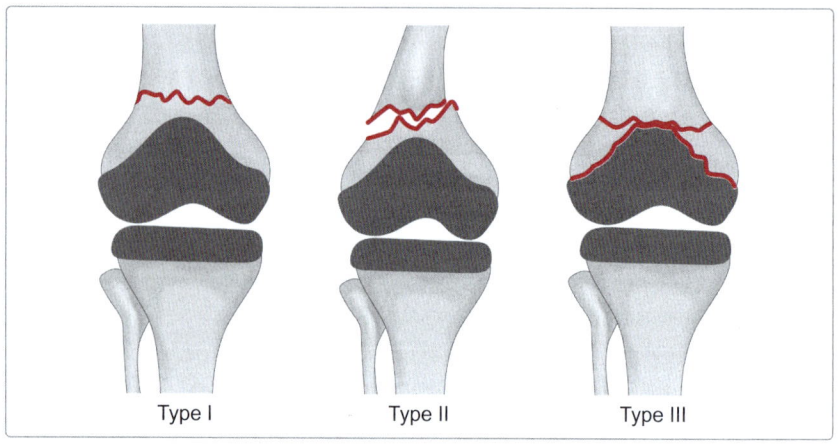

Tibia

Felix Classification
- *Type 1:* Tibial plateau
- *Type 2:* Adjacent to the stem
- *Type 3:* Distal to the stem
- *Type 4:* Tibial tubercle

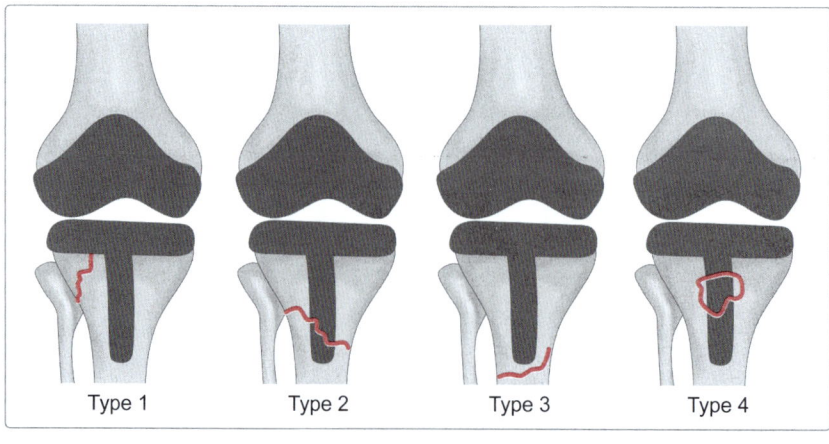

Each has subtypes:
- *A:* Prosthesis well fixed
- *B:* Prosthesis loose
- *C:* Intraoperative

PERIPROSTHETIC INFECTION

Tsukayama Classification
- *Type 1:* Early postoperative
- *Type 2:* Late chronic
- *Type 3:* Acute hematogenous spread
- *Type 4:* Positive intraoperative culture with no clinical infection

LIMB LENGTH DISCREPANCY

Shapiro's Classification
- *Type 1:* The leg length discrepancy increases at a constant rate.
- *Type 2:* It is similar in early to middle childhood but the annual rate of increase diminishes there after.
- *Type 3:* The discrepancy first increases then stabilizes and remains unchanged.
- *Type 4:* Similar to *type 3* in early and middle childhood but then increases toward the end of growth.
- *Type 5:* Consists of an initial increase, stabilizes and then discrepancy decreases.

FUNCTIONAL CLASSIFICATION OF RHEUMATOID ARTHRITIS
- *Class 1:* Patient can perform all daily activities without disability.
- *Class 2:* Patient can perform daily activities with mild discomfort and limited motion at one or more joints.
- *Class 3:* Patient able to perform few duties needed for self-care.
- *Class 4:* Patient is incapacitated. They are bed-ridden or wheelchair bound.

HETEROTOPIC OSSIFICATION OF ELBOW

Hasting and Grahams Classification
- *Class 1:* X-ray evidence of heterotopic bone without functional deficit
- *Class 2:* With functional deficit
  - 2A: Limitation of elbow flexion/extension
  - 2B: Limitation of forearm pronation/supination
  - 2C: Limitation in both planes
- *Class 3:* Ankylosis of joint

OSTEOGENESIS IMPERFECTA (OI)

Looser Classification

- *OI congenita* (presence of numerous fractures at birth)
- *OI tarda* (fractures occur after perinatal period)

Shapiro Classification

- *Congenita A:* Fracture in utero, crumpled femur and ribs (mortality rate: 94%)
- *Congenita B:* Fracture in utero/birth. Normal contour of the bones (mortality rate: 8%)
- *Tarda A:* Fracture before walking age (ambulatory: 67%)
- *Tarda B:* Fracture after walking age (ambulatory: 100%)

Sillence Classification

- *Type I:* Mild, most common form, autosomal dominant inheritance
- *Type II:* Perinatal, lethal
- *Type III:* Progressive deforming
- *Type IV:* Moderate-to-severe
- *Types V:* Similar to type IV in appearance and symptoms of OI, dominant inheritance
- *Types VI:* Extremely rare. It is moderate in severity and similar in appearance and symptoms to OI type IV and is distinguished by a characteristic mineralization defect seen in biopsied bone.
- *Types VII and VIII:* Two recessive types of OI

HEMOPHILIA

Modified Arnold and Hilgartner Classification

- *Stage 1:* Soft tissue swelling
- *Stage 2:* Slight narrowing of the articular space and squaring of bone ends
- *Stage 3:* Marked narrowing of the articular space
- *Stage 4:* Joint disintegration

CHAPTER 10

Diagnostic Criteria

KANAVEL'S SIGN

Criteria for Flexor Tenosynovitis

- Presence of semiflexed position of the involved digit
- Symmetrical swelling around flexor tendon sheath
- Tenderness and erythema along flexor tendon sheath
- Severe pain on passive extension of the digit

KOCHER CRITERIA

Criteria for Acute Septic Arthritis

- Fever
- Inability to bear weight
- Erythrocyte sedimentation rate (ESR) > 40 mm/h.
- Total count > 12,000/mm^3

MORREY AND PETERSON'S CRITERIA

Criteria for Diagnosing Osteomyelitis

- *Definite:* Pathogen isolated from bone or soft tissue, or there is histologic evidence of osteomyelitis.
- *Probable:* A blood culture is positive with clinicoradiological features of osteomyelitis.
- *Likely:* Clinicoradiological features with response to antibiotic therapy.

PELTOLA AND VAHVANEN'S CRITERIA

Criteria for Diagnosing Osteomyelitis

Diagnosis made when at least two of following features are present:
- Pus is aspirated from bone.
- A bone or blood culture is positive.
- Clinical features such as pain, swelling, warmth and limited range of movements.
- Radiological features are present.

RHEUMATOID ARTHRITIS

The European League Against Rheumatism (EULAR) Classification

THE EUROPEAN LEAGUE AGAINST RHEUMATISM (EULAR) CLASSIFICATION	
Symptom duration	**Points**
<6 weeks	0
>6 weeks	1
Joint distribution	
1 large joint	0
2–10 large joint	1
1–3 small joint (with or without)	2
4–10 small joint	3
>10	5
Serology	
RF –ve CRP –ve	0
Low RF +ve, CRP +ve	2
High RF +ve, CRP +ve	3
Acute phase reactant	
Normal ESR or CRP	0
Abnormal ESR or CRP	1

(CRP: C-reactive protein; ESR: erythrocyte sedimentation rate; RF: rheumatoid factor)
Note: Low: <3 × upper limit of normal; High: >3 × upper limit of normal

ANKYLOSING SPONDYLITIS

Rome's Criteria

- Low back pain and stiffness >3 months
- Pain and stiffness of the thoracic region
- Limited motion in lumbar spine
- Limited chest expansion
- History of uveitis

New York Criteria

Clinical Criteria

- Low back pain ≥ 3 months, improved by exercise and not relieved by rest
- Limitation of lumbar spine in sagittal and frontal planes
- Limitation of chest expansion (relative to normal values corrected for age and sex)

Radiological Criteria
- Bilateral grade 2–4 sacroiliitis, or
- Unilateral grade 3–4 sacroiliitis

MIRELS' CRITERIA

Variable	Score*		
	1	2	3
Site of lesion	Upper limb	Lower limb	Trochanter
Size of lesion	Less than 1/3rd	1/3rd–2/3rd	More than 2/3rd
Type of lesion	Blastic	Lytic	Mixed
Pain	Mild	Moderate	Severe

Criteria used to predict fracture risk in long bones in patients with metastasis.

*Score of 8 or more suggest prophylactic internal fixation.

SPINE AT RISK

It denotes increased risk of developing severe kyphosis in patients with TB spine.

Radiological Signs
- Retropulsed diseased segment
- Toppling of the vertebrae
- Facet joint dislocation
- Lateral translation of the vertebrae

Children younger than 7 years of age, with three or more affected vertebral bodies in the thoracic or thoracolumbar spine and two or more "at-risk signs", are likely to have progression of the kyphosis with growth and therefore, should undergo surgical correction.

JUVENILE RHEUMATOID ARTHRITIS (JRA)

International League of Associations for Rheumatoid Arthritis described eight types of JRA:
1. Systemic arthritis
2. Oligoarthritis
3. Extended oligoarthritis
4. Polyarthritis (RF –ve)
5. Polyarthritis (RF +ve)
6. Psoriatic arthritis
7. Enthesitis-related arthritis
8. Other arthritis

Criteria for Diagnosis

- Onset before age of 16 years
- Presence of chronic arthritis > 6 weeks
- Exclusion of other condition by history and laboratory investigations

DIFFUSE IDIOPATHIC SKELETAL HYPEROSTOSIS

Resnick and Niwayama Criteria

- The presence of calcification and ossification along the anterolateral aspect of at least four contiguous vertebral body.
- The presence of relative preservation of intervening disk height in the involved vertebral segment.
- The absence of apophyseal joint bony ankylosis and sacroiliac joint erosion, sclerosis or intra-articular osseous fusion.

NEUROFIBROMATOSIS

Diagnostic Criteria

- At least six café-au-lait spots (>5 mm in children, 15 mm in adults)
- At least two neurofibroma (NF) or one plexiform neurofibroma
- Axillary freckling
- At least two hamartomas in the iris (Lisch nodules)
- Optic gliomas
- Skeletal lesions such as pseudarthrosis of tibia, scoliosis
- A positive family history of NF1 or NF2

SPINE INSTABILITY

White and Panjabi Criteria

WHITE AND PANJABI CRITERIA	
Variable	Score*
Anterior elements destroyed	2
Posterior elements destroyed	2
Sagittal plane translation >3.5 mm	2
Sagittal plane rotation > 11°	2
Positive stretch test	2
Spinal cord damage	2
Nerve root damage	1
Abnormal disk narrowing	1
Dangerous loading anticipated	1

*A score of 5 or more denotes instability.

Diagnostic Criteria

MULTIPLE MYELOMA

The International Myeloma Working Group (IMWG) criteria for diagnosis of multiple myeloma:
- *CRAB (end-organ damage):*
  - *Hypercalcemia:* Serum calcium > 1 mg/dL higher than the upper limit
  - *Renal insufficiency:* Creatinine clearance < 40 mL/min or serum creatinine > 2 mg/dL
  - *Anemia:* Hb > 20 g/L below the lowest limit of normal, or Hb < 100 g/L
  - *Bone lesions:* One or more osteolytic lesion on skeletal radiography, CT, PET/CT

Any one or more of the biomarkers of malignancy (myeloma defining events):
- 60% or greater clonal plasma cells on bone marrow examination
- More than one focal lesion on MRI that is 5 mm or greater in size
- *Serum involves:* Uninvolved free light chain ratio; of 100 or more.

The presence of at least one of these markers is considered sufficient for a diagnosis of multiple myeloma, regardless of the presence or absence of symptoms or CRAB features.

FAT EMBOLISM

Gurd and Wilson's criteria

Major Features
- Respiratory insufficiency (hypoxemia: $PaO_2 < 60$; $FiO_2 = 0.4$, pulmonary edema)
- Cerebral signs (CNS depression)
- Axillary and subconjunctival petechiae

Minor Features
- Pyrexia
- Tachycardia
- Retinal embolism
- Jaundice
- Renal involvement
- Renal involvement
- Fat macroglobulinemia

The presence of one major and four minor features is diagnostic.

Lindeque Criteria

- Sustained $PaO_2 < 60$ mm Hg
- Sustained $PaCO_2 > 55$ kPa or a pH < 7.3
- Sustained respiratory rate > 35 cpm, despite sedation

- *Increased breathing:* Dyspnea, accessory muscle usage
- Tachycardia and anxiety

HYPERLAXITY

Beighton Criteria

This is a screening test for hyperlaxity. The maximum score is 9. A score of 0–3 is considered normal. A score more than 4 indicates laxity.
- *Hyperextension of the 5th MCP beyond 90°:* Left—1, Right—1
- *Apposition of the thumb to the flexor aspect of the forearm:* Left—1, Right—1
- *Hyperextension of the elbow beyond 10°:* Left—1, Right—1
- *Hyperextension of knee beyond 10°:* Left—1, Right—1
- *Able to place palm of both hands on the floor in forward flexion:* 1

Wynne–Davies Criteria

If three of the five pairs of joints examined in any one individual showed this degree of laxity, it is taken as positive.
- Thumb touching forearm on flexing wrist
- Fingers parallel to forearm with wrist extension
- Elbows extend past 180°
- Knees extend past 180°
- Foot dorsiflex past 45°

ADULT RESPIRATORY DISTRESS SYNDROME

According to the 2012 Berlin definition, adult respiratory distress syndrome (ARDS) is characterized by the following:
- Lung injury of acute onset, within 1 week of an apparent clinical insult and with progression of respiratory symptoms.
- Bilateral opacities on chest imaging (chest radiograph or CT) are not explained by other lung pathology (e.g., effusion, lobar/lung collapse, or nodules).
- Respiratory failure is not explained by heart failure or volume overload.
- Decreased PaO_2/FiO_2 ratio (a decreased PaO_2/FiO_2 ratio indicates reduced arterial oxygenation from the available inhaled gas):
  - *Mild ARDS:* 201–300 mm Hg (≤39.9 kPa)
  - *Moderate ARDS:* 101–200 mm Hg (≤26.6 kPa)
  - *Severe ARDS:* ≤100 mm Hg (≤13.3 kPa)

Note that the Berlin definition requires a minimum positive end expiratory pressure (PEEP) of 5 cmH_2O for consideration of the PaO_2/FiO_2 ratio. This degree of PEEP may be delivered noninvasively with CPAP to diagnose mild ARDS.

CHAPTER 11

Formulas in Orthopedics

BIOMECHANICS OF HIP

The power of the abductor muscle should be approximately 2.5 times the body weight to maintain the pelvis level while standing on one leg. The estimated weight on the femur head in the stance phase is the sum of forces created by abductor muscle and body weight which is calculated to be three times the body weight.

$$X \times X\text{-}B = A \times A\text{-}B$$

where,
X = Weight exerted by the body
X-B = Lever arm extending from the body's center of gravity to the center of femur head
A = Abductor force
A-B = Lever arm extending from the center of the femur head to the lateral aspect of greater trochanter

BAUMGARTNER INDEX (TIP-APEX DISTANCE)

This is calculated in cases where an intertrochanteric fracture is being fixed with dynamic hip screw fixation.

It is the sum of the distance between the tip of the lag screw and the center of the head in anteroposterior and lateral view exempting magnification of X-ray. It should be less than 25 mm.

OSTEOTOMY WEDGE

$$W = 0.02 \times \text{Diameter of the bone} \times \text{Correction needed}$$

where,
W = The base of the wedge

For example:
- If elbow is in a varus of 10° due to malunited supracondylar fracture.
- The correction needed is 10 + the normal carrying angle of 10° = 20°.
- Imagine diameter of canal to be 7 mm.
- Hence the wedge = 0.02 × 7 × 20 = 2.8 mm.

CHANGE IN LENGTH AFTER OSTEOTOMY

To determine the change in the length of the limb while doing a varus or valgus osteotomy.

Normally while doing a valgus osteotomy the length increases and while doing a varus osteotomy the length decreases.

$$\Delta H = L (\cos \theta_1 - \cos \theta)$$

where,
H = Change in the length
L = Distance from the middle of the osteotomy to the middle of the femur head
$\cos \theta_1$ = Cosine of the old angle
$\cos \theta$ = Cosine of the new angle

MENELAUS METHOD (LIMB LENGTH DISCREPANCY)

Adolescent older than 9 years; the distal femur grows 9 mm per year and proximal tibia grows 6 mm per year, and growth ceases at 14 years for girls and 16 years in boys.

Menelaus method:
- Calculate current discrepancy
- Calculate the change in discrepancy per year
- Calculate the time remaining for growth
  - *Girls:* 14–current
  - *Boys:* 16–current
- Calculate the discrepancy at maturity:
  Current discrepancy + (Years remaining × Discrepancy per year)

CALCULATION OF NAIL SIZE (PEDIATRIC)

The nail must fill 80% of the narrowest portion of the canal. For example, in a child with femur shaft fracture, if the plan is to put titanium elastic nailing system (TENS): Imagine the narrowest diameter is 9 mm. 80% of 9 mm = 7.2 mm

Hence size of each TENS is 7.2/2 = 3.6 mm, thus in the above case we would be using two 3.5 mm size TENS.

ILIZAROV LENGTHENING

Ilizarov lengthening is started 1 week after corticotomy.

Lengthening is done at a rate of 1 mm/day divided into four sessions of 0.25 mm each.

For example:
If the gap is 4 cm, we have to distract it for 40 days and then if sufficient regenerate is identified on X-ray then the frame has to be kept for double the regenerate time for consolidation, i.e., 80 days.

Hence for a gap of 4 cm, number of days on the frame = 40 + 80 = 120 days.

TIBIAL TUBEROSITY INDEX

It determines the amount of tibial tuberosity to be debrided in Osgood–Schlatter disease.

$$\text{Tibial tuberosity index} = \frac{\text{Distance of B}}{\text{Distance of AB}}$$

where,
B = Distance from the top of the tibial tuberosity to the parallel line of anterior tibial cortex
AB = Top of the tibial tuberosity to the tibial midline

RADIAL BOW CALCULATION

Schmitz and Richards

- It is used to determine the amount and site of maximum radial bow.
- A line is drawn from the bicipital tuberosity to the most ulnar aspect of the radius at the wrist (A).
- A perpendicular is drawn from the point of maximum radial bow to this line.
- The height of the perpendicular (defined as maximum radial bow) is measured in millimeters.
- The distance from the bicipital tuberosity to the previously measured perpendicular at the point of maximum radial bow is then measured and is recorded as a percentage of the length of the entire bow (B).

$$\text{Percentage of radial bow} = \frac{B}{A} \times 100$$

INSALL–SALVATI INDEX

The ratio of the length of the patella tendon : diagonal length of patella. Patella alta is likely if the ratio is > 1.2.

TOURNIQUET PRESSURE

- *Upper limb:* Systolic pressure + 75–100 mm Hg
- *Lower limb:* Systolic blood pressure + 150 mm Hg
- *Width of cuff:* 20% greater than diameter of arm, 40% greater than circumference of thigh

FLEXIBILITY INDEX (SCOLIOSIS)

This is to calculate the flexibility of the curve:

Flexibility index =

$$\frac{\text{Cobb's angle on PA} - \text{Cobb's angle on bend film}}{\text{Cobb's angle on PA}} \times 100$$

TUBERCULOSIS SPINE (CALCULATION OF FINAL DEFORMITY)

This formula was mentioned by Rajasekaran and Shanmugasundaram. This can predict the deformity at 5-year follow-up with fair level of accuracy.

$$Y = a + b \times X$$

where,
Y = Final deformity in degrees at 5-year follow-up
a = 5.5 (constant)
b = 30.5 (constant)
X = Pretreatment vertebral body loss

CHAPTER 12

Radiological Lines

SHOULDER

Gothic arch: Lines drawn along the lateral border of scapula and the medial border of humeral shaft forms an arch resembling roman churches named Gothic arch. This radiological evaluation is done often after shoulder replacement surgeries.

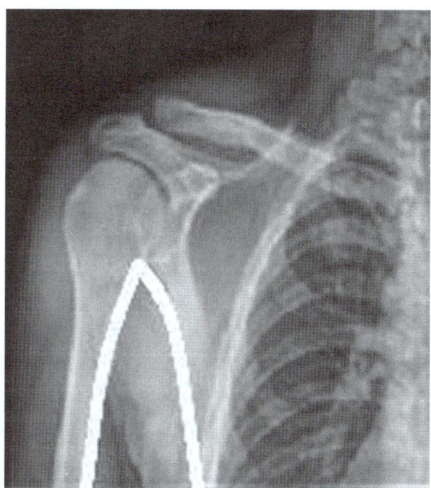

Anteroposterior (AP) X-ray of shoulder showing gothic arch.

Acromioclavicular joint (ACJ): The inferior borders of distal clavicle and acromion should line up. If there is a step, think ACJ injury:
- *Acromioclavicular (AC) distance >8 mm:* AC ligament rupture
- *Coracoclavicular (CC) distance >13 mm:* CC ligament rupture.

Special shoulder X-ray views:
- *Y view:* Orthogonal view of the anteroposterior (AP) shoulder view to view profile of the scapula
- *Grashey view/True AP view:* To view the glenohumeral joint
- *West point axillary view:* Useful in identifying anterior glenoid abnormalities (Bankart lesion)
- *Stryker notch view:* Aimed at assessing posterior humerus (Hill-Sachs lesion)

- *Velpeau view:* Modification of the axillary lateral X-ray of the shoulder intended to be taken with the acutely injured shoulder still in a sling without abduction
- *Garth view:* Tangential view to the shoulder used in trauma to assess the glenoid
- *Zanca view:* To assess the AC Joint
- *Serendipity view:* To assess the sternoclavicular joint and medial one-third of clavicle
- *Supraspinatus outlet view:* To assess AC arch.

ELBOW

Anterior fat pad sign: It is a small radiolucent shadow adherent to the anterior aspect of the distal humerus. An abnormal anterior fat pad is described as a "*sail sign*" because it is unusually prominent and bows outward to form a triangular shape due to hematoma collection indicating an intra-articular fracture.

Posterior fat pad sign: Radiographic visualization of a posterior fat pad is never normal and always signifies fluid in the intra-articular space. This strongly implies fracture of the articular surface.

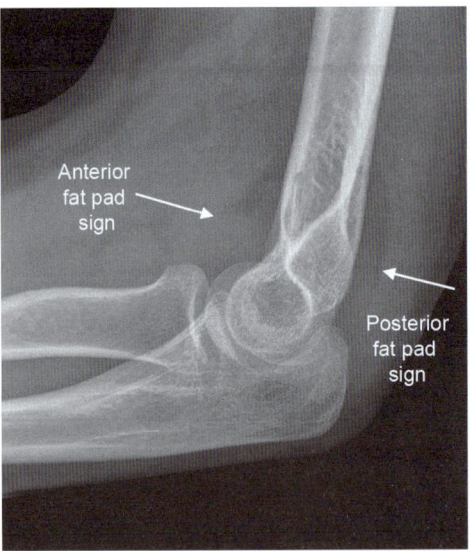

X-ray showing anterior and posterior fat pad signs.

Anterior humeral line: This line drawn along the anterior cortex of the humerus should intersect the middle third of the capitellum on the lateral view. If the film is not a true lateral, interpretation of the anterior humeral line becomes fallible.

Radiocapitellar line: The line drawn through the center of the radius and parallel to it must pass through the capitellum in all degrees of flexion, in all projections.

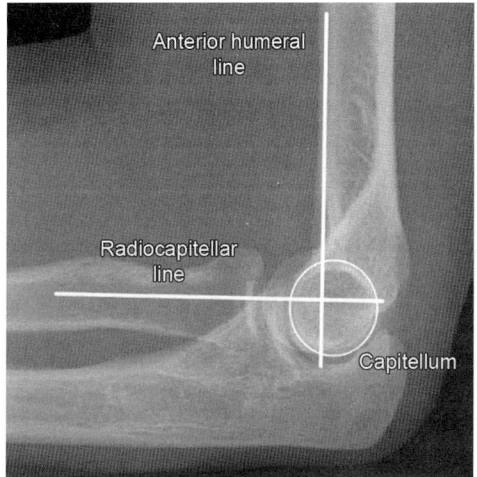

X-ray showing anterior humeral and radiocapitellar lines.

Baumann's angle: It is also known as the humeral-capitellum angle, is used for the evaluation of the displacement of pediatric supracondylar humeral fractures. It is measured on a frontal radiograph, with elbow in extension. This angle is formed by the humeral axis and a straight line through the epiphyseal plate of the capitulum. A value between 64° and 81° is considered normal.

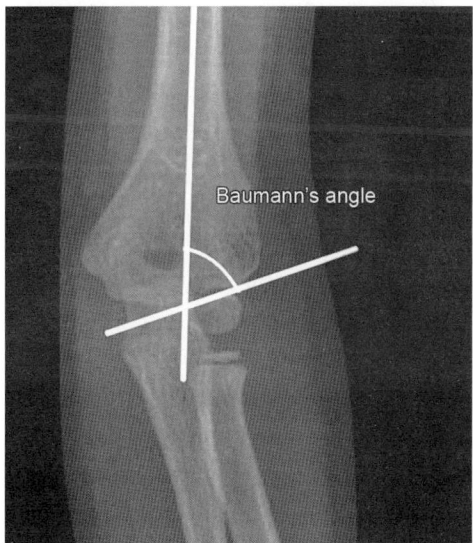

X-ray showing the Baumann's angle.

Shaft condylar angle: On a lateral elbow X-ray, a line is drawn along the long axis of the humerus shaft and another line along the long axis of the humerus condyle. The intersection of both the lines should produce an angle of 30–40°.

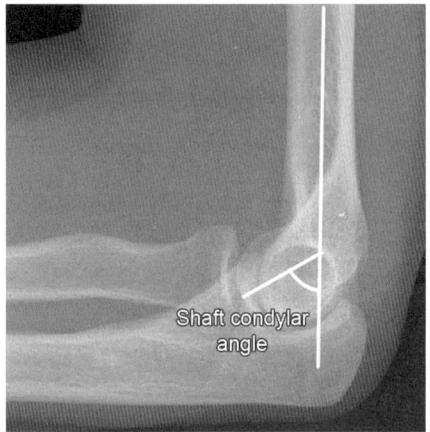

Lateral x-ray of elbow showing shaft condylar angle.

Carrying angle: The angle formed by the humeral axis and the ulnar axis with elbow in extension. Normal carrying angle in males is 8–11° and in females 10–13°. Carrying angle reduces in cubitus varus and increases in cubitus valgus.

Metaphyseal-diaphyseal angle: The metaphyseal-diaphyseal angle is formed between the long axis of the humerus and a line connecting the lateral and medial epicondyles. This ranges from 72 to 95°.

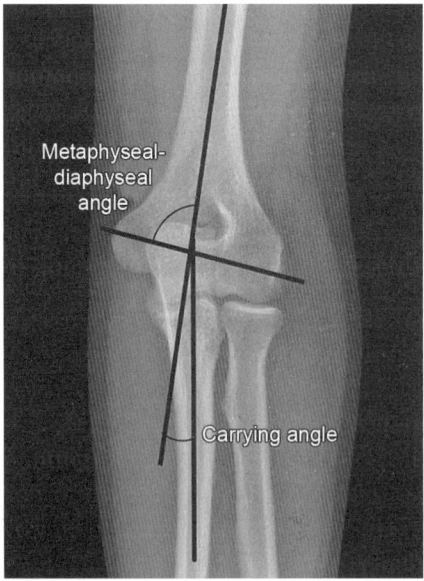

X-ray showing metaphyseal-diaphyseal angle and carrying angle.

Tear drop: It is formed by the coronoid fossa anteriorly and posteriorly by the olecranon fossa. It is broken in case of supracondylar fractures.

Special views: Greenspan view (Radiocapitellar view)—to visualize radial head occult fractures.

WRIST

The articular surfaces of the carpal bones should be parallel and the joint spaces should be about 2 mm wide. Any change in joint space or the shape of a carpal bone may indicate subluxation or dislocation.

Three smooth carpal arcs are formed on the neutral PA view along the radiocarpal and midcarpal joints:
- *Arc 1* follows the proximal surfaces of the scaphoid, lunate and triquetrum.
- *Arc 2* is along the distal surfaces of these same carpal bones.
- *Arc 3* follows the curvature of the proximal surfaces of the capitate and hamate.

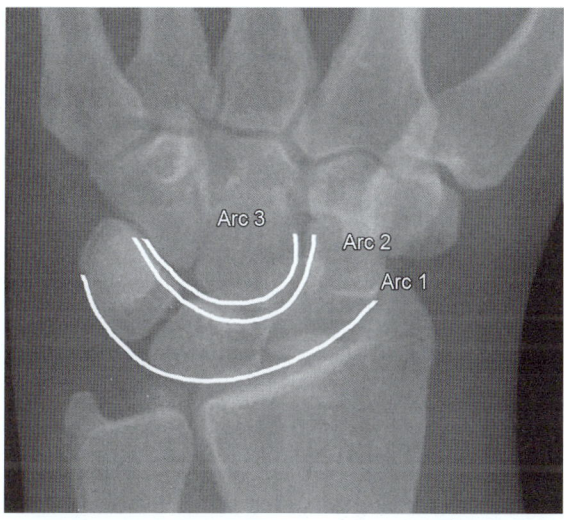

Mnemonic for order of carpal bones in wrist: **S**he **L**ooks **T**oo **P**retty, **T**ry **T**o **C**atch **H**er.

Proximal row: **S**caphoid, **L**unate, **T**riquetral, **P**isiform.

Distal row: **T**rapezium, **T**rapezoid, **C**apitate, **H**amate.

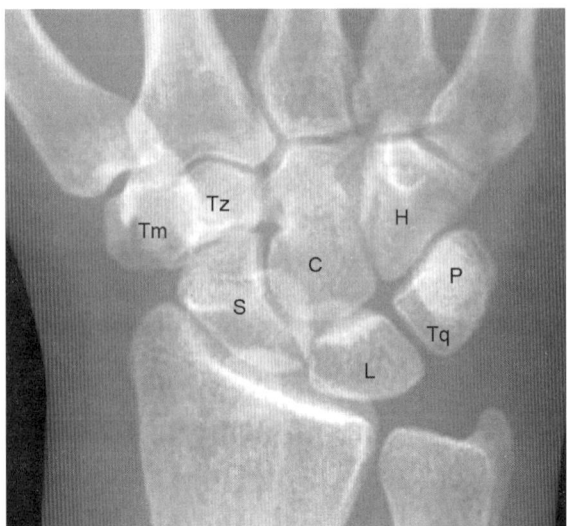

Proximal and distal rows.

Scapholunate dissociation: Increased space between the scaphoid and lunate on a PA film > 4 mm between the scaphoid and lunate (Normal is < 2 mm) is considered pathognomonic for SL dissociation. Widening on X-ray is also termed the *Terry Thomas sign*.

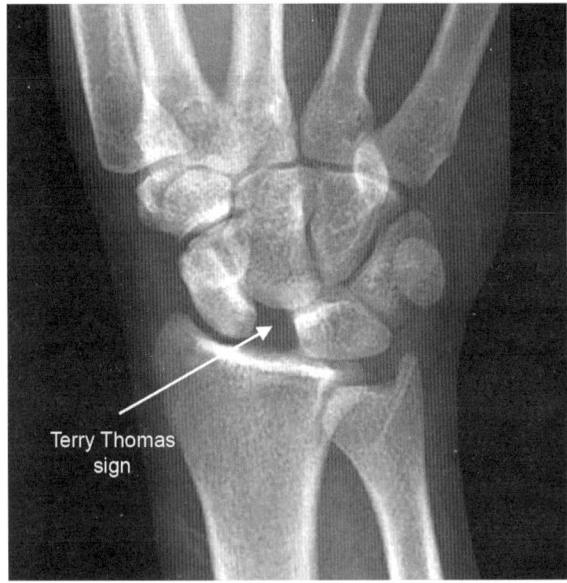

X-ray showing the Terry Thomas sign.

Perilunate instability:
- *On anteroposterior (AP) view:* Break in Gilula's arc, *piece-of-pie sign* (triangular appearance of lunate due to palmar rotation from dorsal force of carpus).
- *On lateral view:* SL angle >70°, *spilled teacup sign*.

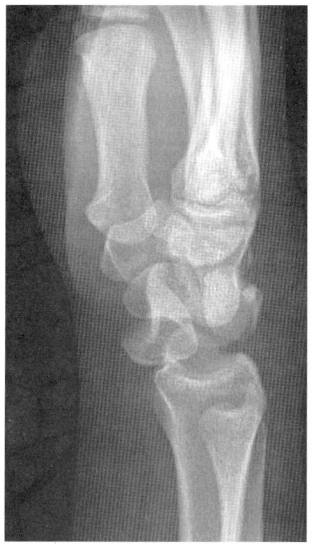 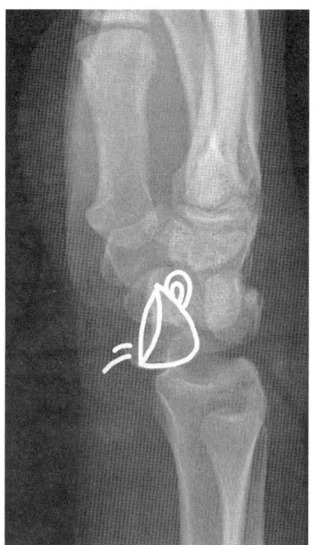

X-ray showing perilunate instability.   X-ray showing spilled teacup sign.

Radial inclination: It is the angle formed by the radial articular surface in AP X-ray to a perpendicular drawn to the radial axis. Normal radial inclination is 22°.

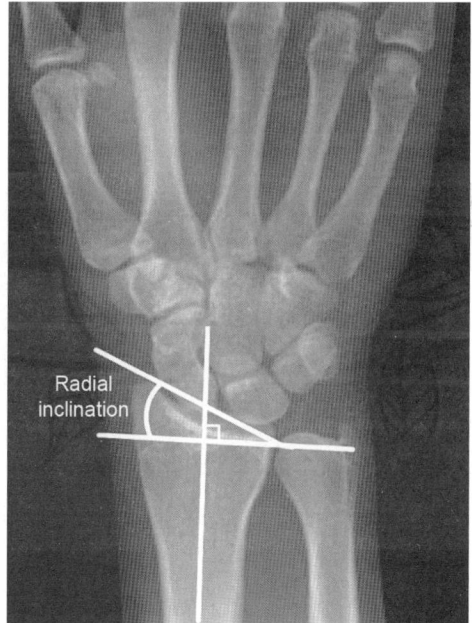

X-ray showing radial inclination.

Radial height: It is a measurement between two parallel lines that are perpendicular to the long axis of the radius. One line is drawn on the articular surface of the radius, and the other is drawn at the tip of the radial styloid. The normal radial height is around 1.2 cm.

Ulnar variance: The difference between the radial articular and ulnar articular surface. Normally it is within 2 mm.

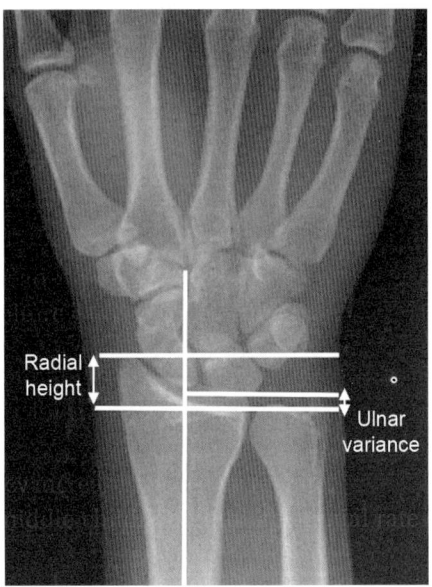

X-ray showing radial height and ulnar variance.

Volar tilt, or volar inclination, is measured on the lateral view. A line perpendicular to the long axis of the radius is drawn, and a tangent line is drawn along the slope of the dorsal-to-volar surface of the radius. The normal angle is 10–25°.

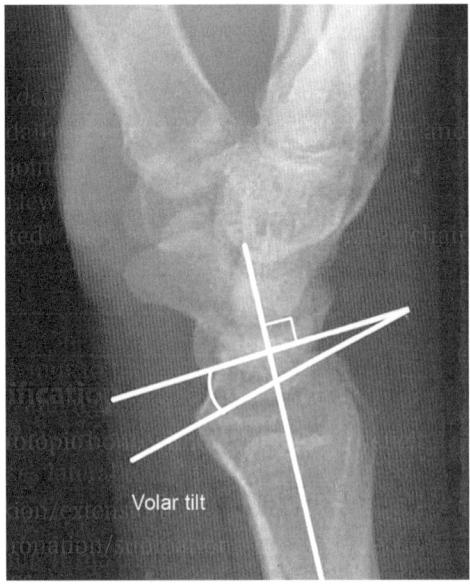

X-ray showing volar tilt.

The **Graham's criteria** are described in **Table 1**.

TABLE 1: Graham's criteria.

View	Measurement	Normal	Acceptable criteria
AP	Radial height	13 mm	<5 mm shortening
	Radial inclination	23°	Inclination >15°
	Articular step off	Congruous	<2 mm step off
Lateral	Volar tilt	11	Dorsal angulation < 5° or within 20° of contralateral distal radius

HIP

True AP pelvis X-ray:
- Pubic symphysis and coccyx are in straight line in middle of screen with 1–3 cm between superior pubic symphysis and tip of coccyx.
- Greater and lesser trochanters should be clearly distinguishable.
- Obturator rings are symmetric.
- *Sacroiliac joint space:* 2–4 mm, equal bilaterally
- Pubis symphysis gap < 5 mm

Iliopectineal/Iliopubic line: The iliopectineal line is the border of the iliopubic eminence. It can be defined as a compound structure of the arcuate line (from the ilium) and pectineal line (from the pubis). With the sacral promontory, it makes up the linea terminalis. The Iliopectineal line divides the pelvis into the pelvis major (false pelvis) above and the pelvis minor (true pelvis) below. Iliopectineal line is disturbed in anterior column fractures of the acetabulum.

Ilioischial line: It is broken in posterior column fractures of the acetabulum.

Tear drop: True floor of acetabulum corresponds to the radiographic teardrop. It lies in the inferomedial portion of the acetabulum, just above the obturator foramen. The lateral and medial lips correspond to the external and internal acetabular walls, respectively; the medial wall is a relatively constant radiographic finding and is not significantly distorted by small degrees of rotation. Tear drop gives an accurate assessment of how much medialization is necessary to have the acetabular component in total hip replacement.

Shenton's line: It is a curve drawn along the inferior border of the superior pubic rami which must trace along the medial neck and shaft of the proximal femur. In case of hip dislocation, proximal migration of femur this line will be broken.

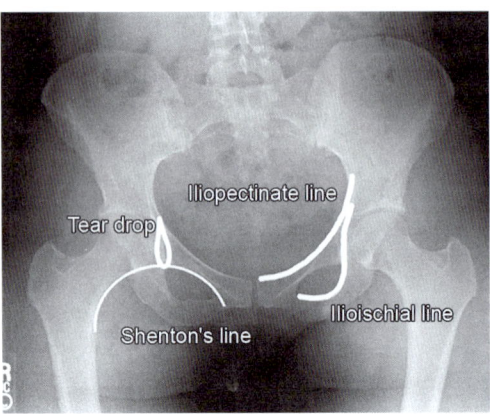

AP X-ray of pelvis showing iliopectineal/iliopubic line, ilioischial line, tear drop, and Shenton's angle.

Acetabular depth: On an AP pelvic radiograph, the relationship of the floor of the fossa acetabuli and the femoral head should be evaluated relative to the ilioischial line. Hips are classified as coxa profunda if the floor of the fossa acetabuli touches or is medial to the ilioischial line, and as protrusio acetabuli if the medial aspect of the femoral head is medial to the ilioischial line.

Tönnis angle/Acetabular index can be determined by drawing three lines on the AP pelvic radiograph:
1. A horizontal line connecting the base of the acetabular teardrops
2. A horizontal line parallel to line 1, running through the most inferior point of the sclerotic acetabular sourcil
3. A line extending from point I to a point L at the lateral margin of the acetabular sourcil (the sclerotic weight-bearing portion of the acetabulum).

The Tönnis angle is formed by the intersection of lines 2 and 3.

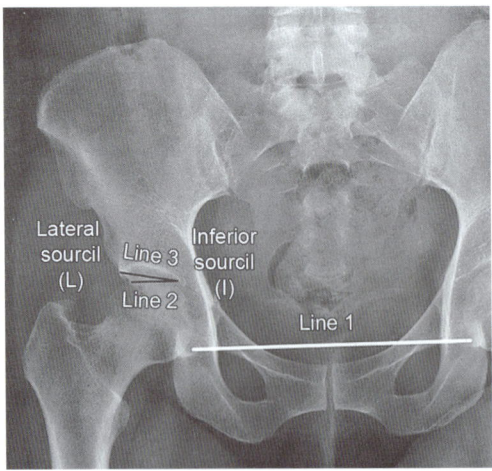

X-ray showing acetabular depth and acetabular index.

Acetabular version: Acetabula can be labeled as retroverted or anteverted on the basis of the presence or absence of a crossover or figure-of-eight sign. An acetabulum is considered to be anteverted if the line of the anterior aspect of the rim does not cross the line of the posterior aspect of the rim before reaching the lateral aspect of the sourcil, and retroverted if the line of the anterior aspect of the rim does cross the line of the posterior aspect of the rim before reaching the lateral edge of the sourcil.

Center-edge angle, a line is drawn through the center of the femoral head, perpendicular to the transverse axis of the pelvis. A second line is drawn through the center of the femoral head, passing through the most superolateral point of the sclerotic weight-bearing zone of the acetabulum. The angle created by the intersection of these two lines is the enter-edge angle. Values of <25° may indicate inadequate coverage of the femoral head.

Head sphericity: On an AP pelvis X-ray using a Mose template (concentric circles) as a reference, if the femoral epiphysis extends beyond the margin of a reference circle by more than 2 mm, the femoral head is considered aspherical.

Neck shaft angle: The angle made by the long axis of the neck of femur and the shaft. In adults it is normally 127° ± 5°. In newborns it is 145°. When the angle is less than 110° it is called coxa vara. When it is more than 140° it is called coxa valga.

Waldenström sign: Distance between medial femoral head and lateral aspect of teardrop. It is a nonspecific indicator for joint effusion. Abnormal if >2 mm difference from contralateral hip.

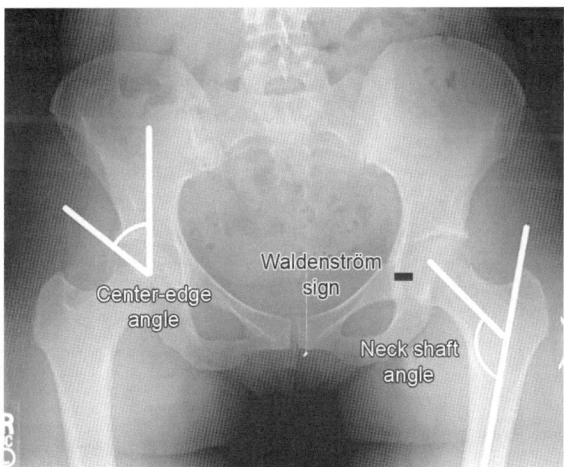

X-ray showing center-edge angle, head sphericity, neck shaft angle, and Waldenström sign.

Perkin's line: It is a line drawn vertical at the outer edge of the acetabular lip.

Hilgenreiner line: It is a horizontal line along the both tear drop/triradiate cartilage.

Hilgenreiner epiphyseal angle (HE angle) is the angle subtended between a horizontal line connecting the triradiate cartilage and the epiphysis); normal angle is <30°.

Klein's line: A line drawn along the superior border of the neck must pass through the lateral part of the head. In case of SCFE it does not pass through the head (Trethowan sign).

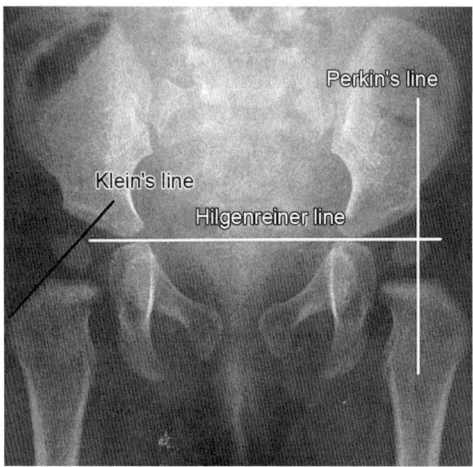

X-ray showing Perkin's, Hilgenreiner, and Klein's lines.

Risser sign: The Risser sign is an indirect measure of skeletal maturity, whereby the degree of ossification of the iliac apophysis by X-ray evaluation is used to judge overall skeletal development. Mineralization of the iliac apophyses begins at the anterolateral crest and progresses medially toward the spine. *Grade 1:* 25%, *Grade 2:* 50%, *Grade 3:* 75%, *Grade 4:* 100% (almost cessation of growth), *Grade 5:* 100% with fusion of apophysis to the iliac crest.

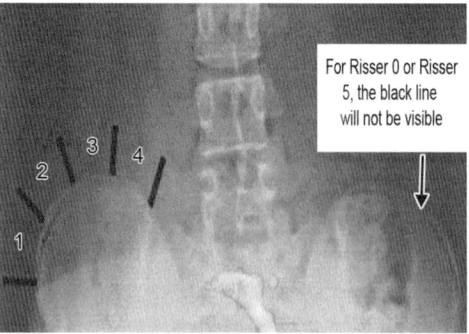

X-ray showing Risser sign.

Schams sign: The inferomedial portion of the femoral neck overlies the posterior wall of the acetabulum inferomedially. This superposition creates a dense triangular appearance on X-rays. Most patients with slipped epiphysis show loss of this dense triangle.

The **metaphyseal blanch sign of Steel** is a crescent-shaped area of increased density, that overlies the metaphysis adjacent to the physis on the AP radiograph. It is caused by superposition of the femoral neck and the posteriorly displaced capital epiphysis.

Singh index:
- *Grade 1:* Only thin principal compression trabeculae visible
- *Grade 2:* Principal compression trabeculae present, other trabeculae nearly resorbed
- *Grade 3:* Principal tensile trabeculae thinned and breakage in continuity present
- *Grade 4:* Principal tensile trabeculae thinned without loss of continuity
- *Grade 5:* Principal tensile and compressive trabeculae readily visible with prominence of Ward triangle
- *Grade 6:* All trabeculae visible and of normal thickness grade 3 and below indicate definite osteoporosis.

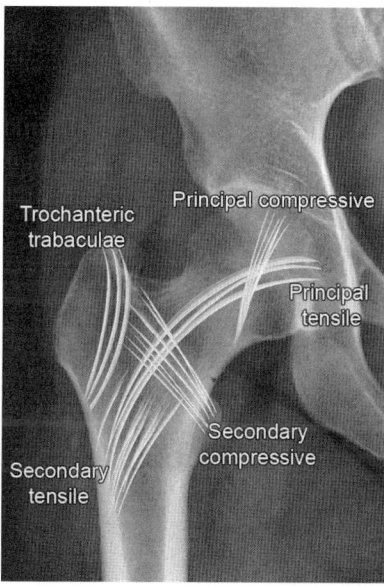

X-ray showing Singh index.

Mechanical axis: A line drawn from the center of the head of femur to the center of talar dome must pass through the knee joint. It makes an angle of 3° from the vertical axis. In genu varum the mechanical axis passes medial to the knee joint and in genu valgum the mechanical axis passes lateral to the joint.

Anatomical axis: It is a line drawn along the shaft of the femur. It makes an angle of 9° with the vertical axis and 6° with the mechanical axis. The normal tibiofemoral angle is 6.85°.

Clinically to assess the alignment of the lower limb the ASIS, center of patella and 2nd toe must be in one line.

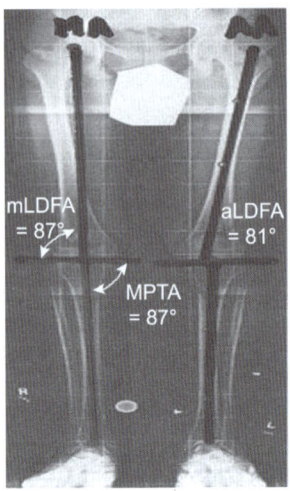

Scanogram of bilateral lower limb showing mechanical axis (MA) and anatomical axis (AA).

KNEE

Quadriceps angle (Q angle): It is formed by the lines connecting the center of patella with the anterior superior iliac spine and center of the tibial tuberosity distally with the patella centered over the trochlear notch (knee should be in 30° flexion). Q angle will be more for females. Increase in Q angle increases the lateral forces on patella. Normal Q angle is 10–14° in males and 15–17° in females.

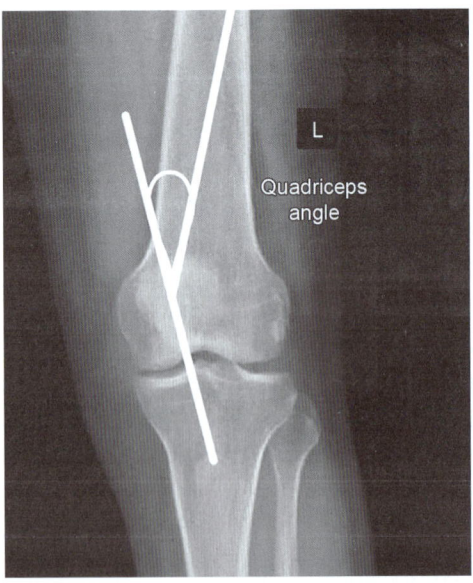

X-ray showing quadriceps angle.

Tibiofemoral alignment: On an AP/PA image, draw a vertical line along the lateral femoral condyle. If the line is more than 5 mm lateral of the lateral tibial plateau, it could indicate a lateral tibia plateau fracture.

Schöttle's point: The Schöttle's point is determined on the lateral view by a line extending from the posterior cortex and another perpendicular to the first, just proximal to the posterior most point of the Blumensaat's line. The Schöttle's point is 1 mm anterosuperior to the intersection of these two lines. It is the point of insertion for MPFL reconstruction.

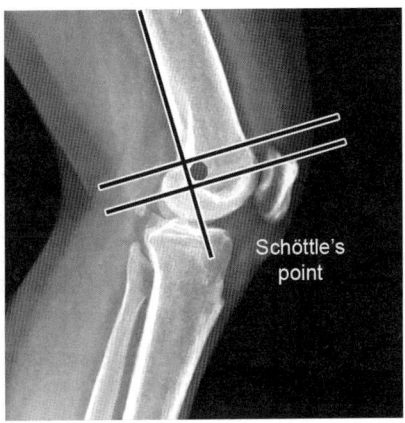

X-ray showing Schöttle's point.

Blumensaat's line: The lower pole of the patella should lie on a line projected anteriorly from the intercondylar notch on the lateral radiograph with the knee flexed to 30°. In cases of patella alta the lower pole will be at a higher level than the line. In patella baja the line might pass through the middle or upper third of the patella.

Insall-Salvati index: It is measured on the lateral knee radiograph with knee flexed to 20–30°. It is the ratio of the longest diameter of patella in lateral view to patella tendon length. Normal range is 0.8–1.2. In patella baja it is <0.8 and patella alta it is >1.2.

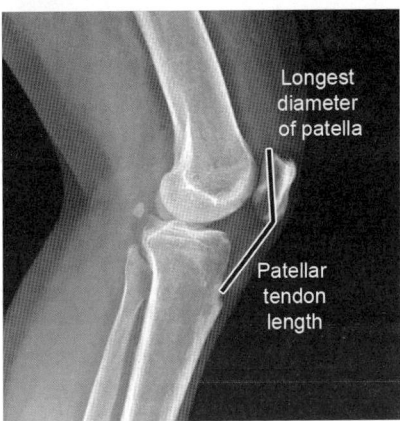

X-ray showing the Insall-Salvati index.

Modified Insall-Salvati ratio: The patellar tendon is measured up to the lower pole of the articulating portion of the patella. The patellar length includes the articulating portion of the patella. The mean normal value ratio is 1.25 and a ratio > 2.0 indicates patella alta.

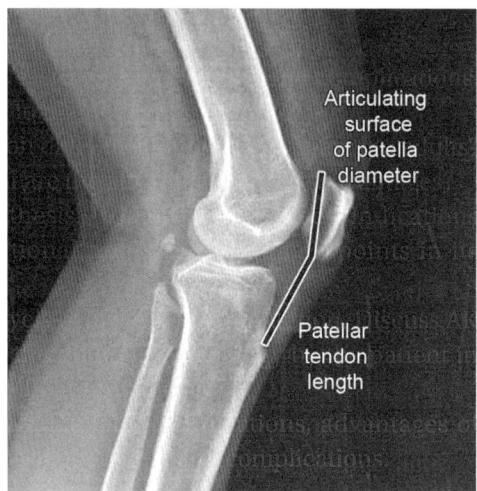

X-ray showing modified Insall-Salvati ratio.

Caton-Deschamps index:
- *Line A:* Distance between the anterior angle of the tibial plateau, to the most inferior aspect of the patellar articular surface.
- *Line B:* Patellar articular surface length.

Caton-Deschamps index = A/B; Normal range: 0.6–1.3; Patella alta: > 1.3; Patella baja: < 0.6

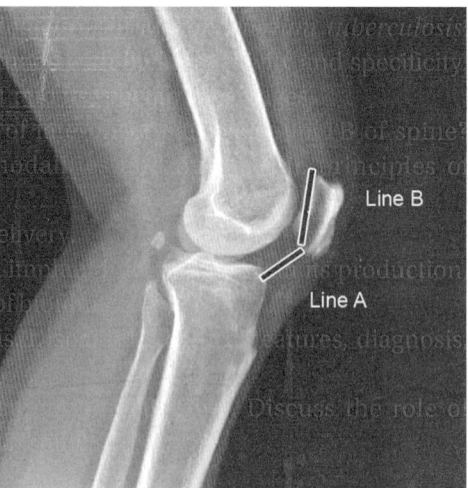

X-ray showing the Caton-Deschamps index.

Blackburne-Peel index:
- *Line A:* Along the patellar articular surface.
- *Line B:* Distance between the horizontal line and the inferior aspect of the patellar articular surface.

B/A is Blackburne-Peel index;
Normal: 0.8; Patella baja: <0.5; Patella alta: >1.0

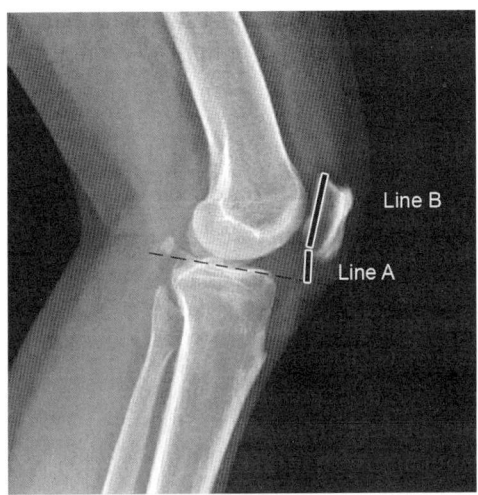

X-ray showing the Blackburne-Peel index.

Sulcus angle: It is formed by the trochlear opening of the knee, measuring the angle between the medial and lateral facets performed at 30–45° of flexion. Its normal value is 135 ± 10°. When the angle of the groove is >145–150°, trochlear dysplasia can be diagnosed.

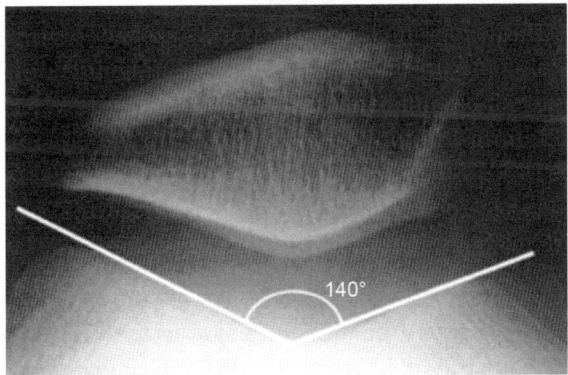

X-ray showing sulcus angle.

de carvalho index:
- *Line A:* The shortest distance between the tibial plateau and the most inferior aspect of the patellar articular surface.
- *Line B:* Patellar articular surface length.

de Carvalho index = A/B; Patella alta: >1.11

TT:TG distance: Superimpose axial images of femoral condyles and tibial tuberosity.

Draw a line along the posterior femoral condyles, and then draw the following lines perpendicular to this line:
- Bisecting the tibial tuberosity (TT)
- Bisecting the trochlear groove sulcus (TG)
- Measure the distance between TT and TG = TT-TG distance—normal: <15 mm; borderline: 15–20 mm; abnormal: >20 mm.

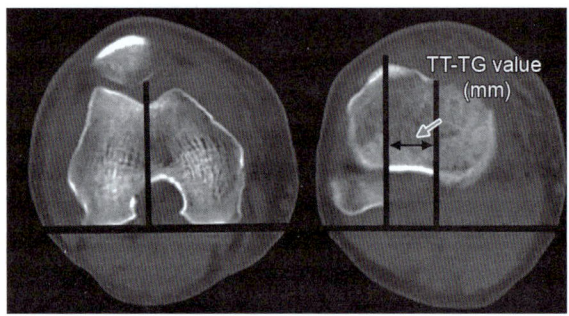

X-ray showing the TT:TG distance.

Special knee X-ray views:
- *Merchant view:* Superior-inferior projection of the patella.
- *Laurine view:* Inferior-superior projection of the patella.
- *Rosenberg's view:* Weight-bearing projection in 45° knee flexion used to assess joint space-related pathology such as osteoarthritis.

ANKLE

Tibiofibular clear space: The interval between the medial border of the fibula and the lateral border of the posterior tibial malleolus on ankle mortise radiograph is normally 6 mm or less. Increase indicates syndesmotic injury.

Tibiofibular overlap of <10 mm on AP ankle radiograph is indicative of syndesmotic injury.

Talocrural angle: It is measured on AP radiograph with a line drawn parallel to articular surface of distal tibia and line connecting tips of both malleoli (intermalleolar line); this angle is normally 83° ± 7°. It helps in assessment of restoration of fibular length.

Talar tilt: Difference of more than 2 mm in AP X-ray in the superior clear space on the medial and lateral aspect is indicative of a positive talar tilt.

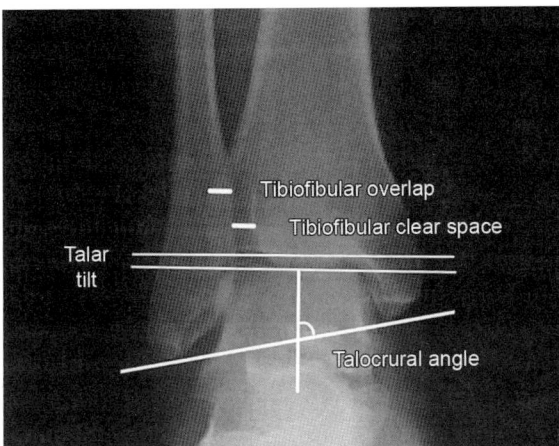

X-ray showing tibiofibular clear space, tibiofibular overlap, talocrural angle, and talar tilt.

Talar shift: Increase in medial or lateral clear space >1 mm indicates talar shift.

Bohler's angle: The angle between line from highest point of anterior process to highest point of posterior facet plus line tangential to superior edge of tuberosity; measured on lateral foot X-ray. Normally 20–40°.

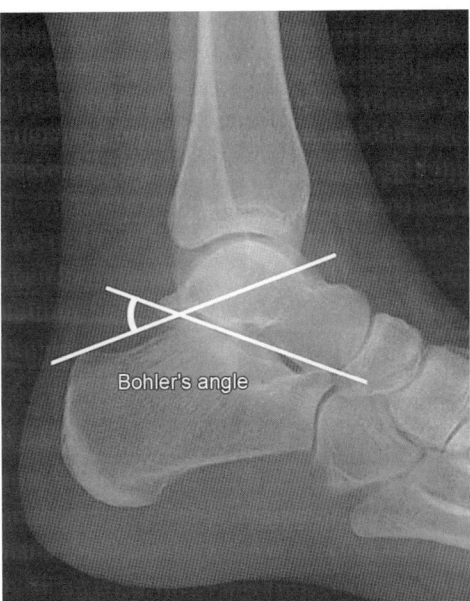

X-ray showing the Bohler's angle.

Tibiocalcaneal angle: It is measured on the lateral ankle X-ray. It is the angle formed by the long axis of tibia and the long axis of calcaneum. Normal angle is 70°.

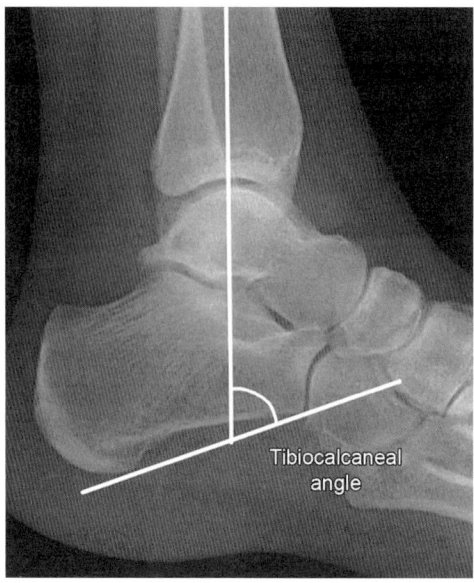

X-ray showing tibiocalcaneal angle.

Tibiotalar angle is the angle between the talar neck axis and the tibial anatomic axis. Normal value around 65–70°.

Gissane's angle: The angle formed between the posterior and middle facet is the critical angle of Gissane. Normal Gissane angle is between 95° and 105°.

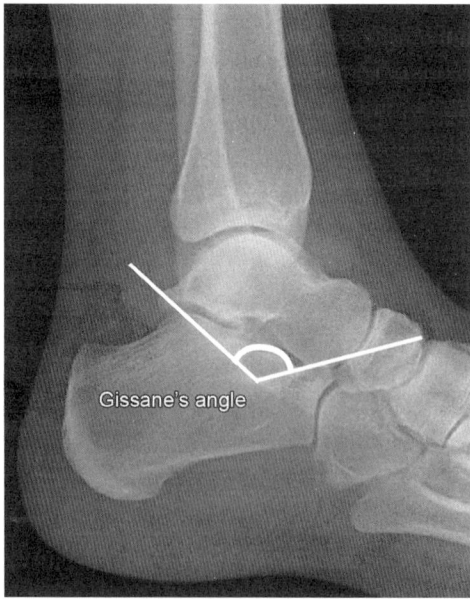

X-ray showing Gissane's angle.

Special ankle views:
- *Mortise view* done with the leg internally rotated 15–20° so that the X-ray beam is perpendicular to the intermalleolar line. This view permits examination of the articular clear space.
- *Broden view:* Used to better visualize the subtalar joint.
- *Canale view:* Best view to demonstrate talar neck fractures.

FOOT

First-second intermetatarsal angle: The angle formed between the first and the second metatarsals is normally less than 10°. In metatarsus primus varus, the angle is more than 10. This angle is important to decide on the choice of osteotomy for hallux valgus correction.

Hallux valgus (HV) angle: The angle formed between the first metatarsal and the proximal phalanx of Hallux. It is normally less than 15°. It is more in case of hallux valgus.

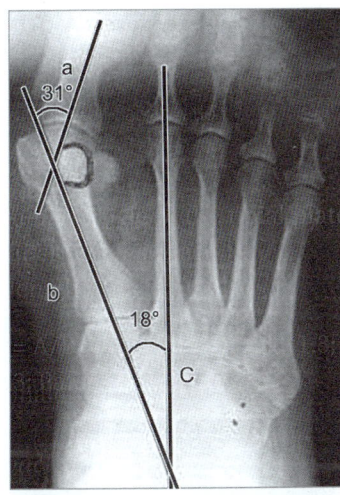

AP X-ray of foot showing intermetatarsal angle and hallux valgus (HV) angle.

Hallux interphalangeal angle is the angle formed between the intersection of the longitudinal axes of proximal phalanx and the distal phalanx of the hallux. Normal value 11°.

AP Meary's angle: It is the angle between a line drawn from the centers of longitudinal axes of the talus and the first metatarsal. It is used to identify the apex of deformity in patients with pes cavus and pes planus on lateral weight-bearing foot radiographs. Normal value is around 5–10°.

Lateral Meary's angle: Angle formed by the bisection of the talar neck axis and the anatomic axis of the first metatarsal. Normal value is around 6°.

Talocalcaneal angle (Kite's angle): The angle formed between the tangent drawn along the inferior border of the calcaneus and the long axis of the talus. In newborn the angle is 25–55°. In adults it is 30–50°. In hindfoot valgus the angle is more than 55° and in hindfoot varus it is less than 30°.

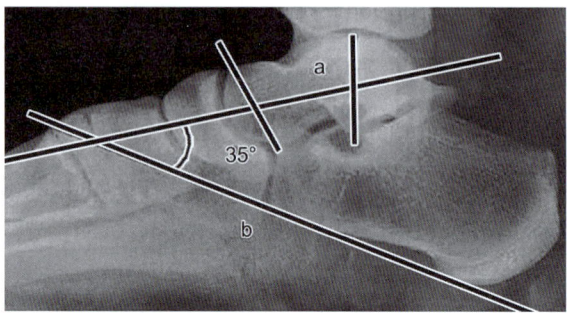

Lateral X-ray of foot showing Kite's angle.

SPINE

- *A:* It is a smooth curve along the posterior aspect of the spinous process of all cervical vertebrae.
- *B:* It is a line drawn lamina of all vertebra (spinolaminar line).
- *C:* It is line drawn along the posterior vertebral border.
- *D:* It is line along the anterior vertebral border.
  All lines have to be uniform indicating appropriate alignment.

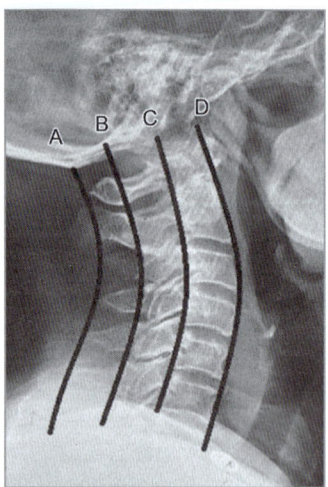

Lateral X-ray of cervical spine showing orientations of the lines.

Atlantodens interval (ADI) is <3 mm in adults or <5 mm in children, Basion-dens space is <12 mm.

- *A* shows the retropharyngeal space in the upper cervical area. It is about 7 mm anterior to C2 vertebra.
- *B* denotes the retropharyngeal space along the lower cervical spine. In front of the C6 vertebra the retropharyngeal space measures about 20 mm.

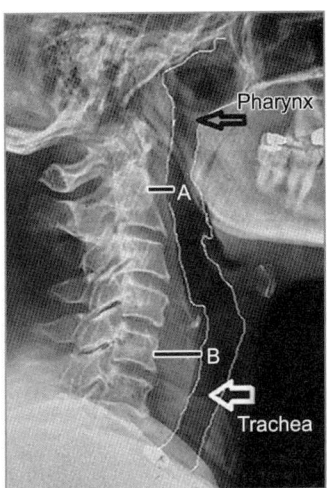

Lateral X-ray of cervical spine showing difference in measurement of retropharyngeal space at different levels.

Torg ratio: It determines the presence of spinal canal stenosis.

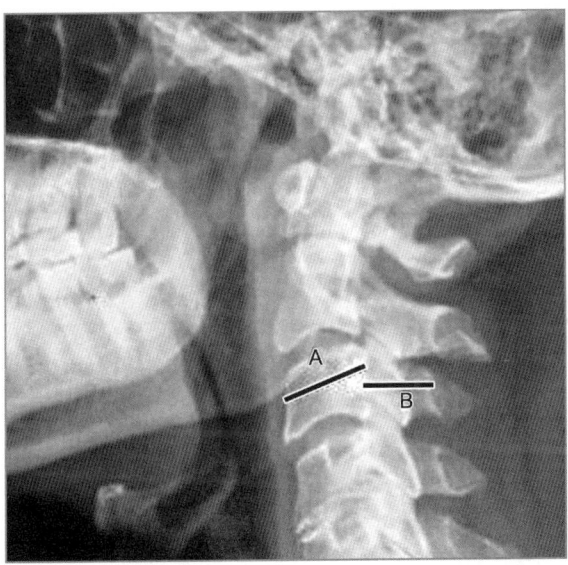

Lateral X-ray of cervical spine showing Torg ratio.

It is the ratio of the spinal canal diameter to the vertebral body diameter in lateral view.

A ratio <0.8 indicates significant spine stenosis and increased risk of neurological injury.

$$\text{Torg ratio} = B/A$$

Powers ratio identifies anterior or posterior atlanto-occipital subluxation.

$$\text{Powers ratio} = BC/OA$$

BC is the distance from the basion to the midvertical portion of posterior laminar line of the atlas. OA is distance from opisthion to midvertical portion of posterior surface of anterior arcus of the atlas.

Chamberlain line: It helps to determine basilar invagination.

It is the line joining the posterior aspect of the hard palate with the posterior rim of the foramen magnum on the lateral view; if the tip of dens is >3 mm above this line, invagination is present.

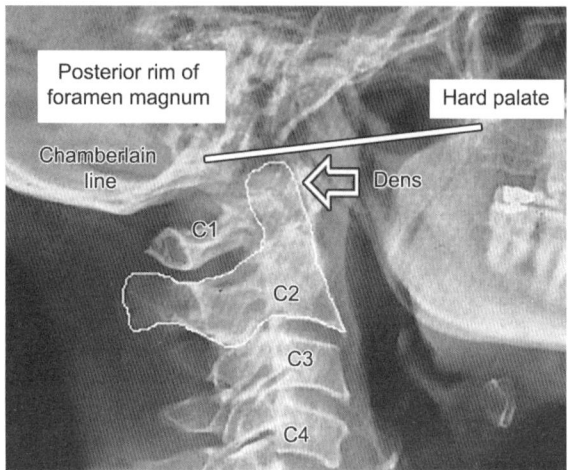

Lateral X-ray of cervical spine showing Chamberlain line.

McGregor line: This line is a modification of the Chamberlain line and is used to determine basilar invagination when the opisthion is not identified on plain radiographs.

It is a line connecting the posterior edge of the hard palate to the most caudal point of the occipital curve.

If the tip of the dens lies more than 4.5 mm above this line it is indicative of basilar invagination.

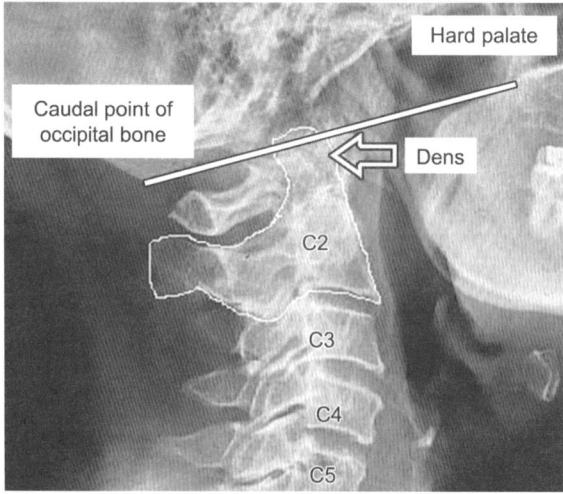

Lateral X-ray of cervical spine showing McGregor line.

McRae line: It is a line drawn to determine basilar invagination. A line is drawn from the anterior border to the posterior border of the foramen magnum.

The dens is normally 5 mm below this line. If the tip of dens migrates above this line it is indicative of atlantoaxial impaction.

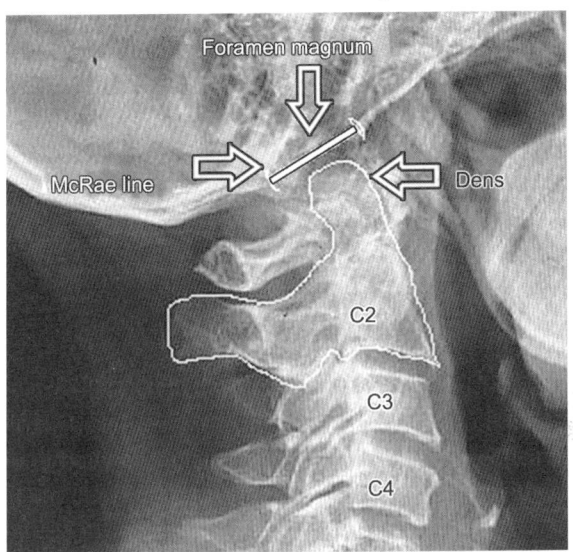

Lateral X-ray of cervical spine showing McRae line.

Wackenheim line: This is a line drawn from the caudal extension of the dorsal surface of the clivus and is used to measure the distance of space to the tip of the dens (or odontoid process).

Bimastoid line: This is described to evaluate basilar invagination on the AP view.

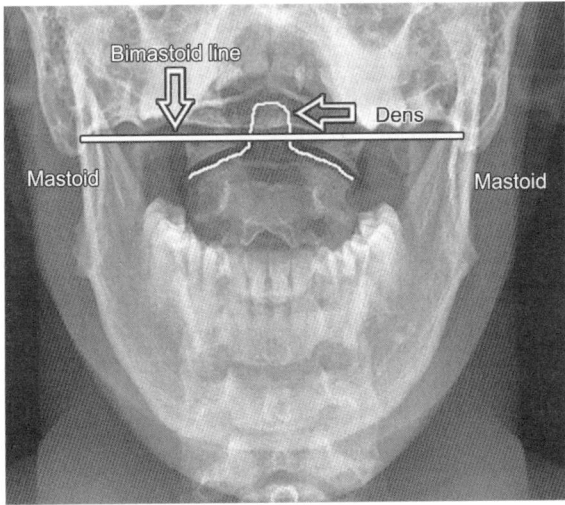

X-ray of open mouth view showing bimastoid line.

The bimastoid line is drawn between the inferior tips of the mastoid bilaterally. The tip of the C2 normally projects less than or equal to 10 mm above this line.

Basilar invagination is present when the tip of the odontoid process projects above 10 mm.

Digastric line: This is a line connecting the right and left digastric grooves on a coronal cut of a CT scan or AP skull radiograph. It is used to measure the distance from the tip of the dens (odontoid process) to help evaluate the presence of a basilar invagination. The tip of the dens should be around 11–12 mm below this line.

Kyphosis can be measured by the **Cobb method** on the lateral X-ray.

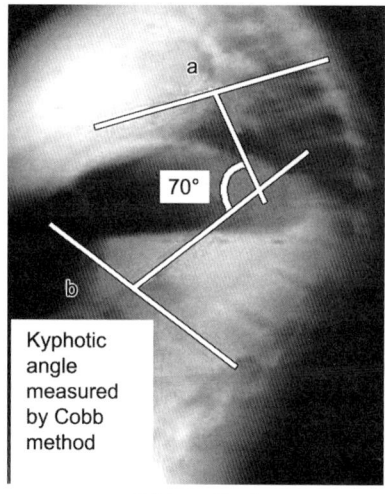

Cobb method.

The angle is made between the line tangential to the upper end plate of the upper most vertebrae and the lower end plate of the lower most vertebrae.

The normal thoracic kyphosis is 30–50°. The normal kyphosis is measured between T4 and T12.

Plumb line: Normally a plumb line drawn from the occiput in the midline must pass through the spinous process of all vertebrae and the mid sacrum. Any deviation from midline is indicative of scoliosis. This X-ray shows a neutral or balanced scoliosis, i.e., even though there is deviation of vertebrae from midline the plumbline from occiput passes through the sacral midline. This X-ray shows a thoracolumbar scoliosis with right convexity extending from T4 to L2.

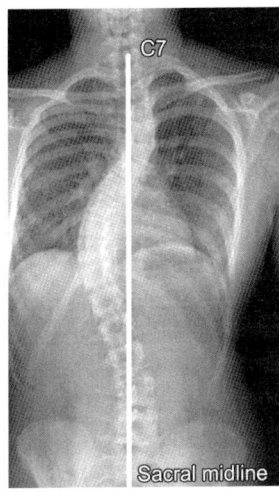

X-ray showing scoliosis and plumb line.

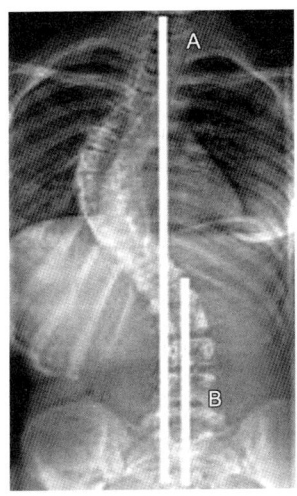

X-ray showing thoracolumbar scoliosis.

Positive scoliosis: In this X-ray the scoliosis is to the right side. The plumbline dropped from occiput also passes lateral to the sacral midline on the right side. When the plumbline passes lateral to the sacral midline on the side as that of the convexity, it is called positive scoliosis. When the plumbline passes on the opposite side as that of the scoliosis, it is called negative scoliosis.

Cobb method: It is a method to measure the scoliotic angle.

The angle is between the tangent drawn to the superior end plate of the superior most vertebrae and the inferior end plate of the inferior most vertebra.

The inferior and superior vertebrae are the one that is tilted into the curve. Apex vertebra is the vertebra which is maximum deviated from the midline on the convex side of scoliosis.

Indirect Cobb angle: When perpendicular lines are drawn from the two tangential lines to measure the Cobb angle as shown in the X-ray.

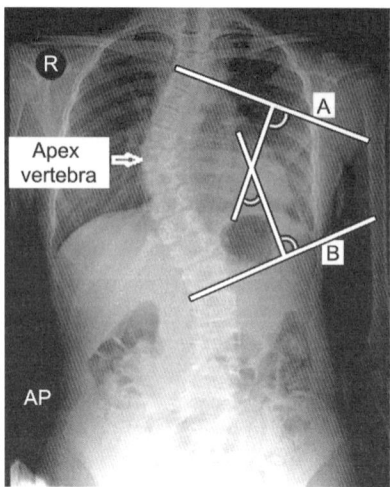
Indirect Cobb method.

Rib vertebral angle difference (RVAD) of Mehta: It is calculated by subtracting the angle of the rib on the convex side of the curve relative to the line perpendicular to the vertebral body end plate from the angle on the concave side of the curve. In this X-ray:, A-B is the RVAD. RVAD > 20° is associated with significant risk of progression.

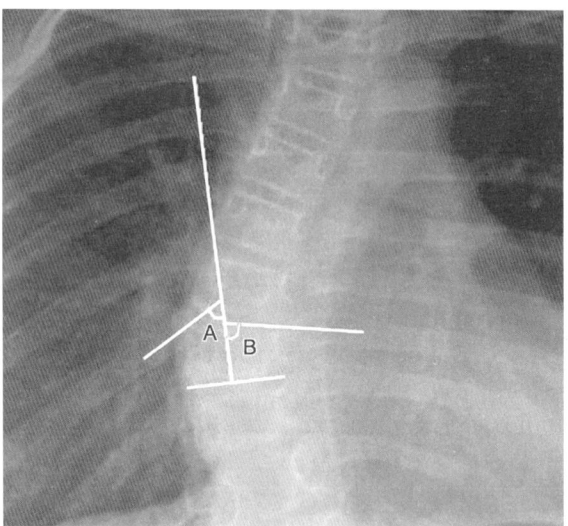
X-ray showing rib vertebral angle difference (RVAD).

Scottish Terrier: Oblique views are routinely taken to evaluate spondylolisthesis. In normal oblique view at 45° the posterior elements give the image of Scottish Terrier:
- *Transverse process:* Mouth
- *Pedicle:* The eye

- *Superior process:* Ear
- *Pars interarticularis:* Neck
- *Inferior process:* The fore leg
- *Lamina:* The belly
- *Spinous process:* The hind part

Scottish Terrier sign: In spondylolisthesis when there is a pars interarticularis fracture or lysis there will be a defect seen in the neck part (beheading) of Scottish Terrier as shown in the X-ray.

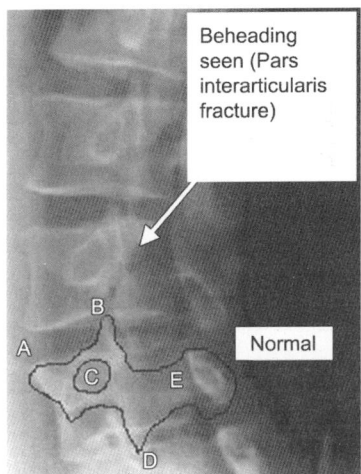

Lateral X-ray of spine showing Scottish Terrier sign.

Percentage of slip: It is measured to evaluate the anterior slip. B is the distance the vertebrae has slipped anteriorly and A is the sagittal diameter of the upper vertebra.

$$\text{Percentage of slip} = B/A \times 100\%$$

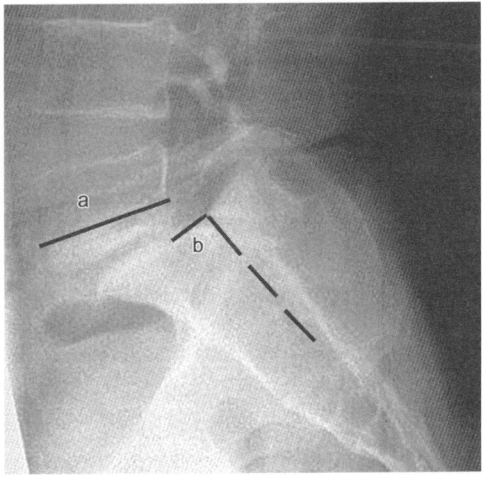

Percentage slip calculation.

Slip angle: The slip angle is measured by drawing a line perpendicular to a line drawn along the posterior aspect of the first sacral vertebral body and measuring angle between that and a line parallel to the inferior endplate of L5. As the slip progresses, area of contact between the L5 and S1 decreases and the body of L5 tilts forward on the sacrum. Preoperative slip angle of more than 35° is risk for slippage. In this X-ray, it is the angle between *a* and *b*.

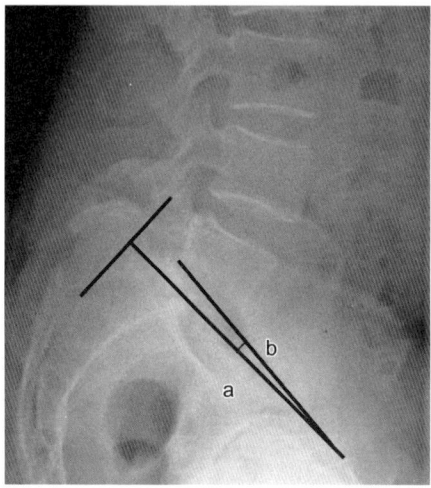

Slip angle calculation.

Sagittal balance: A vertical line (plumb line) is drawn from the middle of the body of the C7 vertebral body. This line should pass through the

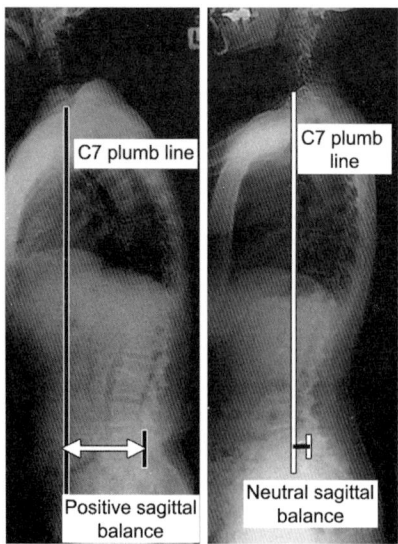

X-ray showing sagittal balance.

superior endplate of S1, or more precisely within 2 cm of the posterosuperior corner of the S1 vertebral body. The position of this line is then termed positive, neutral or negative:
- *Positive balance:* The plumb line passes more than 2 cm in front of the posterosuperior corner of the S1 vertebral body
- *Neutral balance:* The plumb line passes within 2 cm of the posterosuperior corner of the S1 vertebral body.
- *Negative balance:* The plumb line passes more than 2 cm behind the posterosuperior corner of the S1 vertebral body.

Sacral slope: The mean sacral slope is 42° in standing and 30° in sitting position. A line parallel to the sacral end plate is drawn. The angle subtended between this line and the horizontal reference line is the pelvic tilt.

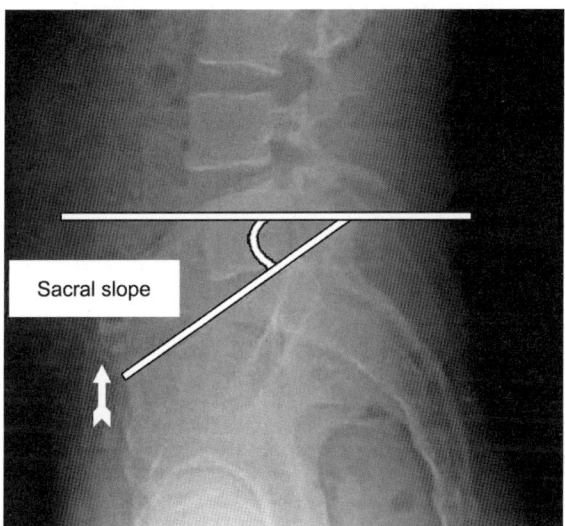

X-ray showing pelvic slope angle.

Pelvic tilt: A line from the midpoint of the sacral end plate is drawn to the center of the femoral heads. The angle subtended between this line and vertical reference line is the pelvic tilt. Normal is 12°.

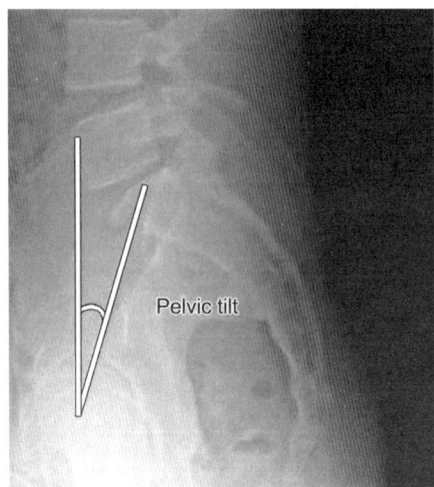

X-ray showing pelvic tilt angle.

Pelvic incidence: The pelvic incidence (PI) is measured as an angle formed by two vectors: The line joining the bicoxofemoral axis to the center of the sacral end plate and a line perpendicular to the sacral endplate. In this image D is the mid-point of the line joining the center of two femoral heads (bicoxofemoral axis). C is the line joining bicoxofemoral axis and the sacral end plate. B is the perpendicular drawn to the sacral end plate.

Pelvic incidence (PI) = Pelvic tilt (PT) + Sacral slope (SS)

Normal pelvic incidence is 50°.

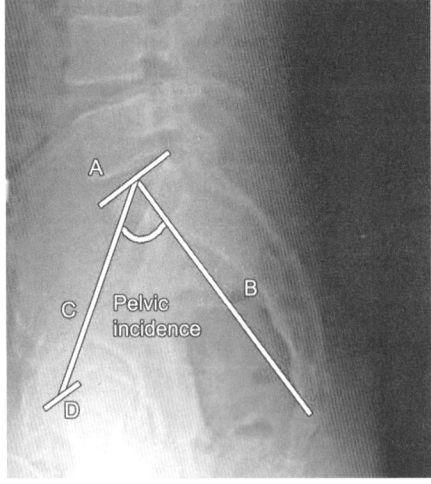

X-ray showing pelvic incidence.

BIBLIOGRAPHY

1. Beaty JH, Kasser JR (Eds). Rockwood & Wilkins' Fractures in Children: Monteggia Fracture-Dislocation in Children, 6th edition; 2006. pp. 477-551
2. Bucholz RW, Heckman JD. Rockwood and Green's Fractures in Adults, 5th edition. Philadelphia: Lippincott Williams and Wilkin; 2001.
3. Buck-Gramcko D. Congenital malformations of the hand and forearm. Chir Main. 2002;21(2):70-101. doi:10.1016/s1297-3203(02)00103-8.
4. Canale ST, Beaty JH. Campbell's Operative Orthopedics, 12th edition. St Louis: Elsevier Mosby; 2008.
5. Herkowitz HN, Garfin MD SR, Eismont FJ, Bell GR, Balderston RA. Rothman-Simeone, The Spine, 5th edition. Philadelphia: Saunders; 2006.
6. Periasamy M, Venkatramani H, Shanmuganathan RS. Management of chronic Achilles Tendon injuries—review of current protocols and surgical options. Indian J Plast Surg. 2019;52(1):109-16. doi:10.1055/s-0039-1687923.
7. Rajasekaran S, Sabapathy SR, Dheenadhayalan J, Sundararajan SR, Venkatramani H, Devendra A, Ramesh P, Srikanth KP. Ganga hospital open injury score in management of open injuries. Eur J Trauma Emerg Surg. 2015;41(1):3-15. doi:10.1007/s00068-014-0465-9. PMID: 2603816.
8. Sabapathy SR, Periasamy M. Healing ulcers and preventing their recurrences in the diabetic foot. Indian J Plast Surg. 2016;49(3):302-13. Doi:10.4103/0970-0358.197238.
9. Tuli SM. Tuberculosis of the Skeletal System, 5th edition. New Delhi: Jaypee Brothers Medical Publishers; 2016.
10. Wolfe SW, Pederson WC, Kozin SH, Cohen MS. Green's Operative Hand Surgery, 16th edition. New York: Elsevier; 2016.

CHAPTER 13: DNB Practical Examination

What to do? (The Authors' Experience and Guiding Points)

As the pandemic occurred, there was also a change in pattern of the Diplomate of National Board (DNB) examinations. From traveling to another state to give your practical examinations, taking long and short cases in limited time, sometimes with the need of a translator, to now having an Objective/Observed Structured Clinical Examination (OSCE) pattern with majority being online, *the pattern of examination conduction has totally changed* and this brings confusion into the minds of students as to what to expect, what to concentrate on and how to prepare for the examination.

Here in this book, we share the experience of how the examination was conducted when the new pattern was first released, how we prepared and how we scored. Read on to know what to expect from the *New DNB Practical Examination* pattern. Actually, a blessing in disguise!

Firstly, have everything in order. Real examiners will be present and hence you need to be upto the mark. A nice clean white coat, an instrument kit, neat haircut and trimmed facial hair, polished shoes and be ahead of time at the examination venue.

The venue will usually be kept in the *same city as the candidate* so as to avoid interstate travel. However, a few unlucky ones may get their center in a bit far off place. National Board of Examination (NBE) was kind enough to ask students, which is their preferred city and for those who were allotted a different place, NBE did change venues on a request basis.

Now Comes the Examination and its Rules

Day of Examination

Observed Structured Clinical Examination pattern for 200 marks: In this, students are provided with a table and chair and 25 sheets of papers. The chairs are all facing one common screen on which NBE will project their questions.

Each question will have subparts, a picture and sometimes even a video. Each OSCE question carries *8 marks* and there are *25 such questions* (hence the 25 sheets of paper).

When the examination begins, each student will be seated at their allotted table and will be watching the screen. NBE streams their questions live to all centers so every student will be seeing the same question at the same time. You have 5 minutes to answer each question (timer will be displayed as well). The questions asked in OSCE are all based from theory mostly, some from orthotics, prosthetics, and some from ward rounds and instruments. But majority questions are from the theory you studied a few months ago. The questions are simple and the subparts can also be vague. Meaning, they can ask you a subquestion which if you want, can answer for 10 marks too, but since you do not have that much time, answer precisely to the point, try to cover as much as you can in the answer, but finish up in time. The examiner is looking for certain keywords in your answer and as long as you hit that, you have got your marks.

For example, an X-ray of a tumor is shown to you and Part A is to identify the tumor which you would be able to answer in a few seconds. Part B would be, discuss its management. You can write a lot regarding its management starting from conservative to limb salvage, however, you do not have that much time and neither do you have that much space. Space? What space? Each sheet provided to you for answering is collected and scanned and sent to NBE as soon as you finish your 5 minutes. And only one side is scanned. Therefore you have only one side of an A4 sheet to write all the answers. And once your 5 minutes is up, that sheet is taken away from you. No second chance to revise your answer!

So read your question carefully and answer all the questions as soon as possible (ASAP) with keywords or flowcharts, whatever best describes your answer, *maximum content in minimum time!* Really, time management is the main game changer in OSCE. Sometimes gait videos will be poorly streamed and you will struggle to make out whether it is a Trendelenburg gait or a short limb gait. Quickly move on to the subquestions and try to answer them rather than spending time trying to figure out why the video is so bad or why they did not get any better video to send!

Therefore in summary, for an OSCE, be prepared with your theory, read the question fast, answer maximum in the 5 minutes with keywords you think are most apt for it and manage your time well. Time management is the key!

Few examples of OSCE questions are listed here so that you can know what types of questions will appear in examination:

Q. A 50-year-old diabetic presented with a swollen finger with fever for 1 day following thorn prick:
A. What is your diagnosis? (2)
B. What are the other three cardinal clinical signs? (3)
C. Who described these signs? (1)
D. How will you treat this patient? (2)

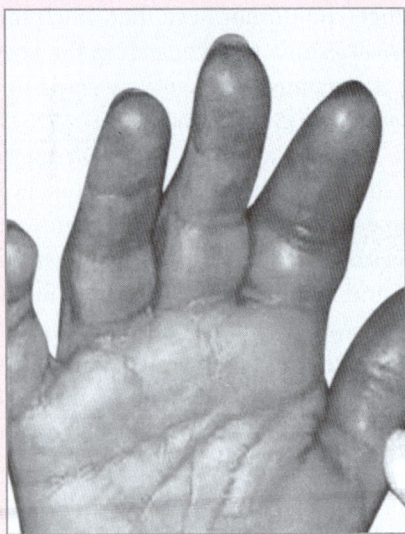

Q. There is a FIRE in the operation theatre in your hospital. You are the first at the scene of the fire:
A. Which emergency code will you activate? (2)
B. What is RACE protocol? (2)
C. What is PASS protocol while using a fire extinguisher? (2)
D. What is the code for a medical emergency? (2)

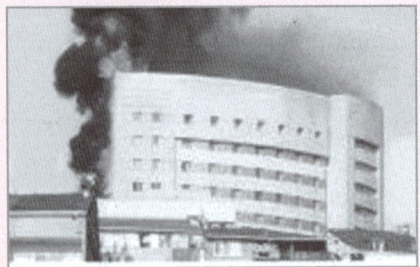

- Define evidence-based medicine (2)
- Schematic representation of levels of evidence pyramid. (6)

Q. A 50-year-old lady with past history of bilateral salpingo-oophorectomy 15 years ago presents with increasing dorsal kyphosis and following report:
A. What is your diagnosis? (1)
B. WHO definition of the above condition. (2)
C. How to classify the above disease as "Severe"? (2)
D. Mention any three drugs categories used for medical management of the disease. (3)

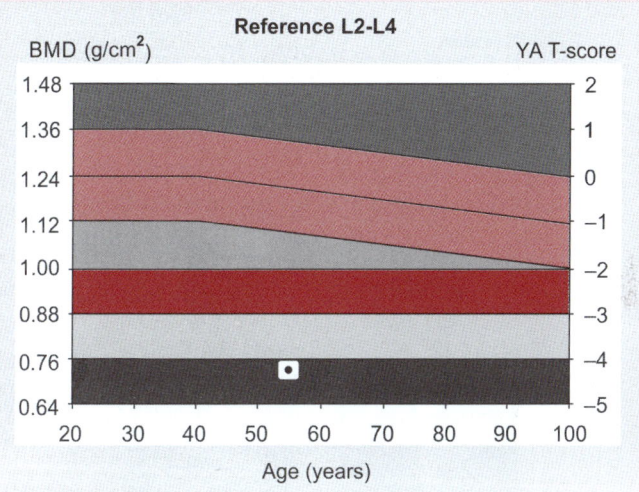

A. Identify the condition? (1)
B. What are the radiological findings? (2)
C. What are the stages of this condition? (3)
D. Treatment modalities. (2)

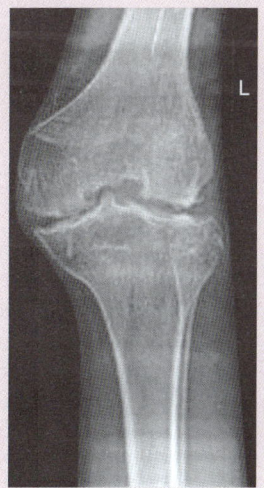

A. Class to which the drug belongs. (1)
B. Classification of the drug class with examples. (2)
C. Indications of use (3)   D. Side effects (2)

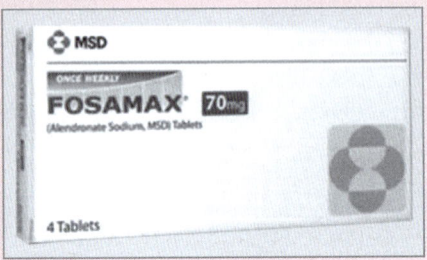

A. Identify (1)   B. Describe (2)
C. What is the principle? (1)   D. Uses (2)
E. What are good prognostic markers for this brace? (2)

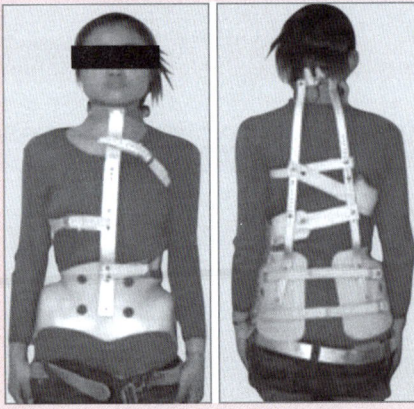

A. Identify the clinical test. (2)
B. Which clinical condition is diagnosed by this test? (2)
C. Clinical signs of the given condition. (2)
D. Pathology of the clinical condition. (2)

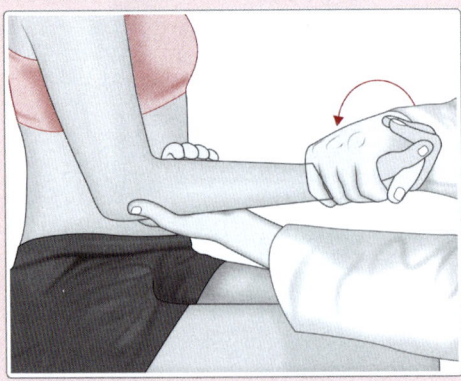

A. Name the contents of the six compartments shown in the figure. (6)
B. Name the pathology which affects the contents of the 1st compartment. (1)
C. What is intersection syndrome? (1)

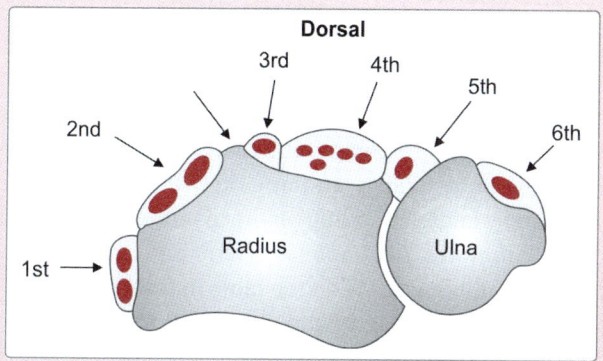

Post OSCE Comes the Clinical Cases and Viva Stations

Clinical Cases

Two cases of 30 marks each will be kept.

One case will be a virtual case shown to you on a laptop streamed from the NBE center while the other case will either be a volunteer patient or a real patient on whom skill demonstration will have to be done. Gone are the days of taking history and examining the patient and findings and reaching a diagnosis.

In the skill demonstration segment, a patient will be made to lie down (could be a real patient or a volunteer) and the examiner will ask you to demonstrate certain tests or certain findings. For example, he could ask you how would you do a Thomas test and what are its interpretations, how will you measure Bryant's triangle, how will you demonstrate a varus/valgus stress test, what is Coleman block test, show me the tests for median nerve and you will have to demonstrate these tests in the right manner and be ready to answer any of the questions the examiner can ask regarding that topic which could include theory also. Hence both in OSCE and in viva, theory knowledge plays a vital role. This session usually lasts for 15 minutes.

In the second station, a virtual case will be provided to you. You will be seated in front of a laptop with the examiner having a laptop too opposite you. Both the laptops will have the same questions, images and case scenario projected on it. The examiner is, however, provided with a set of keywords which the candidate is expected to put in his answers. For example, an image of a leg that has undergone multiple surgeries is provided to you and an X-ray of the same limb showing nonunion of tibia is shown to you. The case history talks about a man who sustained an open fracture and underwent multiple procedures leading to nonunion. The subsequent questions could be what is the classification of open tibia fracture, what is the classification of nonunion, what would you like to do in this case, what findings would you expect in this case, what are the other treatment options, if the patient is not affordable what would you do, etc. The questions would be many and you would have to answer it with a clinical mindset trying to cover all possibilities so that you hit the right words and marks are granted accordingly. There is no time limit here in both the case scenarios.

Besides the two cases, there are four viva stations. One on instruments, one on X-rays, one on osteology and one on orthotics and histopathology. Here anything can be kept depending on the institute's specimen availability. Approximately 5 minutes per table is spent and the examiner can ask anything he pleases about what is on the table in front of him.

This is the general format of the examination. There is no negative marking for the OSCE and there is no case history taking and examination (at least until now, they may change this in forthcoming sessions). Initially, it was necessary to get 50% marks from the total (OSCE + case + viva) to pass, however, they later changed it to 50% in OSCE and 50% in other stations to pass. Things have been kept simple and chances of passing the examination are way higher as compared to before. Of course, the mentality of the examiners cannot be predicted but most often being from the same city, they are usually considerate to their fellow students.

This pattern can have minor alterations as further sessions are conducted especially with the skill demonstration portion where they may even keep a real patient and have a case history taking session. At present, with the pandemic looming, NBE is trying to avoid this but it is still at the discretion of the institution. So keep your eyes open for these changes as NBE is still refining its process of conducting this new modality of examination pattern.

Wish you all the best.

Question Bank

BASIC SCIENCES AND GENERAL ORTHOPEDICS

- Define gait. What are its phases? Enumerate various pathological gaits with their causes.
- Give one example each of concentric and eccentric contractions during gait cycle. How will paralysis of tibialis anterior affect normal gait?
- Define fat embolism syndrome (FES). Describe in brief clinical features, diagnosis, and management of FES.
- Explain callotasis.
- Properties of bone graft. Different types of bone graft, bone graft substitute and their incorporation. Differentiate between cancellous and cortical grafts.
- Differentiate between primary and secondary fracture healing.
- Define and classify VIC. Describe etiopathogenesis, clinical features, prevention, and management of VIC.
- Define compartment syndrome. Describe pathogenesis, clinical features, investigations, and management of acute compartment syndrome of leg.
- Describe the properties of synovial fluid (synovial fluid analysis). How does it help in differentiating various types of arthritis?
- Write a short note on hemophilic arthropathy.
- Explain terrible triad of death (hypothermia, acidosis, coagulopathy).
- Define distraction histiogenesis. Write the principles of distraction histiogenesis.
- Enumerate the indications of distraction histiogenesis in orthopedics.
- Differentiate between antalgic and Trendelenburg gait.
- What is thoracic outlet syndrome? Discuss its anatomy and etiology. How will you diagnose and treat it in OPD?
- Write a short note on Bone Bank.
- Explain allograft and its definition, types, principles of preservation, advantages, and disadvantages.
- Describe in brief the current state of knowledge of use of stem cells in orthopedic practice.
- Describe the stages of fracture healing. List the factors influencing fracture healing. Discuss the physical and chemical modalities to augment fracture healing.

- Explain autologous transfusion.
- Describe gene therapy in orthopedics.
- Describe metabolic acidosis.
- Describe postoperative fever.
- What is pneumatic tourniquet? Discuss its uses, complications, and safety guidelines.
- Define "Virchow's triad" and the management of DVT. What precautions are required if postoperative epidural analgesia is used for 4–5 days?
- What is Kienbock's disease? Write in brief etiology, diagnosis, and management of this disease.
- Describe the musculoskeletal manifestations of sickle cell anemia.
- Describe bone remodeling unit. Briefly describe the drugs which influence remodeling.
- Explain biochemical markers of bone formation and resorption.
- Describe respiratory distress syndrome.
- Write a short note on BMP.
- What is "VAC"? How will you manage a case of compound fracture tibia having no neurovascular deficit?
- Describe physiology of normal articular cartilage and its biomechanical functions. Discuss the advances in articular cartilage tissue engineering and repair.
- Describe chronic (exertional, recurrent) compartment syndrome.
- Describe etiopathogenesis, pathology, and management of DIC.
- Describe blood supply of long bones. Discuss the effects of various modalities of fixation on the blood supply.
- Describe the structure of bone with illustrative diagrams.
- Describe various types of cartilage. Discuss their physiology and ultrastructural characteristics.
- Describe postoperative pain management and patient control analgesia.
- Enumerate bleeding disorders encountered in orthopedic practice. What is hemophilic pseudotumor? Discuss its management.
- Describe gate control theory of pain.
- Describe ATLS.
- What is damage control orthopedics? How will you manage a case of fracture?
- Describe shaft of femur with lung contusion in adult.
- Describe Crush syndrome.
- Describe ARDS.
- Define polytrauma. Explain fluid management and clinical monitoring of polytrauma patient with hemorrhagic shock.
- Describe hypotensive resuscitation.
- Describe Mangled Extremity Severity Score (MESS).
- Describe transfer protocol of completely dismembered finger and limb from site of injury to hospital.

- Explain Ganga scoring.
- Explain clinical features and management of stove-in-chest.
- What is ballistics? Briefly describe the current management of ballistic injuries of the spine.
- Define shock. Explain its pathophysiology of septic shock. Discuss the management of shock in a polytrauma patient.
- Define a "borderline" patient of polytrauma. Discuss the clinical/investigative parameters to decide whether the patient should be managed by Early Total Care (ETC)/Damage Control Orthopedics (DCO).
- What is reperfusion injury? How can we prevent it? Outline the principles of its management.
- Describe the management of multiple rib fracture with hemothorax.
- Describe the methods of reducing risks of blood transfusion.
- What is multiorgan dysfunction syndrome? What are indicators of mortality? Write briefly about diagnosis and management.
- Discuss prophylaxis against secondary complications of patients with polytrauma.
- Describe tension pneumothorax.
- Describe massive blood transfusion.

ARTHRODESIS

- Describe pantalar arthrodesis.
- Give functional classification of muscles around the shoulder. Enumerate the indications for shoulder arthrodesis. What are the prerequisite for good results? Describe any one technique of shoulder arthrodesis.
- Describe Stewart and Harley ankle arthrodesis.
- Describe Bristow's procedure.
- Describe triple arthrodesis for equinus.

ARTHROPLASTY

- Explain types and principles of HTO for OA.
- Define tribology. Describe recent advances in biomaterials in joint replacements to increase their longevity.
- Outline the biomechanical principles of total knee replacement and describe gap balancing technique.
- What is reverse shoulder arthroplasty? How is it different from conventional shoulder arthroplasty? Enumerate the indications and biomechanical basis of design of this prosthesis.
- Enumerate bearing surfaces in total hip arthroplasty (THA). Describe its advantages and disadvantages of each.
- Describe bearing surface.

Question Bank

- Describe recent advances in THA.
- Describe tantalum in arthroplasty.
- Classify periprosthetic fracture following THA. Outline the management strategy.
- Describe the role of PCL in knee arthroplasty. Discuss the benefits of PCL retention versus substitution.
- Describe the role of navigation in total knee arthroplasty.
- Draw diagram(s) of anatomic and biomechanical axis of LL and briefly discuss the biomechanical principles of TKR.
- Enumerate complications of TKR.
- What is highly cross-linked polyethylene? How it is manufactured? How does it affect modern THA?
- Describe the role of templating in THA. Outline the steps of templating in protrusio acetabuli and a lateralized hip with suitable diagrams.
- Describe combined angle of anteversion during THA.
- Describe biomechanics of hip joint and its clinical application.
- Describe the anatomy of PCL. Discuss pros and cons of cruciate retaining versus cruciate sacrificing TKR.
- Describe pathogenesis of medial compartment osteoarthritis. Discuss pros and cons of HTO versus unicondylar replacement.
- Describe the concepts of total knee replacement.
- Describe management of unicompartmental OA knee.
- Discuss the causes of loosening after THA. Discuss its clinical features, diagnosis, and management.
- Discuss differential diagnosis in a 25-year-old male presenting with monoarticular arthritis of knee joint. Tabulate the management in algorithmic manner.
- Discuss various methods of preventing DVT following TKR. Discuss their merits and demerits.
- Describe bone defects encountered during TKR and their management.
- Classify periprosthetic fracture around knee. Outline its treatment strategy.
- Describe anticoagulants in arthroplasty.
- Briefly describe the relevant biomechanics of the lower limb particularly in relation to bone cuts in TKR.
- Describe indications and contraindications of total elbow arthroplasty. What are the complications of total elbow arthroplasty? Explain the changes in design to reduce complications.
- Describe total ankle arthroplasty.
- Describe the principles of surface replacement arthroplasty of hip. What do you think are the reasons of failure of previous historical designs compared to modern successful design?

AMPUTATION

- Describe the early management of closed above knee amputation.
- Describe indications (absolute and relative) and complications of amputation. Explain the principles of amputation of lower limb in children.
- Discuss the principles of amputation in children and adults.
- What is Syme's amputation? Describe its indications and complications. What is the prosthesis suitable for Syme's amputation?
- How do principles of amputation differ in children as compared to adults? What is pylon prosthesis? What are the advantages and disadvantages?
- Describe suction socket prosthesis. Explain its principles, indications and advantages over conventional prosthesis and main points in its construction.
- Enumerate various classical levels of lower limb amputation. Discuss AK amputation in detail. What is the difference in energy by the patient in AK amputation as compared to BK amputation?
- Describe skew flap amputation. Explain its indications, advantages of conventional amputation, steps of operation, and complications.
- Explain ideal stump.

INFECTIONS

- Describe surgical site infection and its prevention and treatment.
- Describe precautions taken by surgical team during operation of HIV positive patient.
- Describe the sequelae of septic hip in an infant.
- Describe the spina ventosa.
- Explain instrumentation in spinal TB with its rationale and indications.
- Explain ATT regimen in bone and joint TB.
- Explain recent advances in detection of *Mycobacterium tuberculosis*. Enumerate various newer methods with their sensitivity and specificity. Describe GeneXpert/CB-NATT and its specific advantages.
- What are the various causes of late-onset paraplegia in TB of spine? Describe the investigative modalities and outline the principles of management.
- Describe the local antibiotic delivery.
- Describe the role of biofilm in implant infection. Explain its production, regulation, and management of biofilm.
- Define Tom Smith hip arthritis. Discuss the clinical features, diagnosis, treatment, and sequelae.
- Describe the indications of surgery in TB spine. Discuss the role of instrumented stabilization in TB spine.

Question Bank

- Write briefly the current presentation and treatment strategy in MRSA infection. Briefly mention about its evaluation.
- Describe the clinical features and complications of TB of cervical spine.
- Explain necrotizing fasciitis.
- Explain COVID-19 in orthopedics.
- Briefly describe the clinical features, diagnosis, differential diagnosis, and broad principles of management of TB dorsal spine with paraplegia.
- Discuss the etiology, pathology, diagnosis, and management of gas gangrene of the lower extremity.
- What is tubercle? Discuss pathoanatomy, diagnosis, and principles of management of cold abscess.
- Describe the mechanism of bacterial colonization and perpetuation in osteomyelitis after orthopedic implant surgery. How is the situation different in TB infection of musculoskeletal system?
- Describe chronic recurrent multifocal osteomyelitis.
- Describe gram-negative septicemia.
- Define osteomyelitis. Discuss the pathology, clinical features, investigations, and management of acute osteomyelitis of upper end of tibia in a 10-year-old child.
- What is tuberculoma? Discuss the primary drug used to treat TB spine.
- Enumerate complications of isoniazid, streptomycin, and ethambutol.
- Define multidrug-resistant TB (MDR TB). Discuss the clinical features, diagnosis, and treatment of a case of MDR TB of spine.
- Describe the clinical features, diagnosis, and management of TB hip of children.
- Explain psoas abscess.
- Define osteomyelitis. Discuss the pathology, clinical features, diagnosis, and management of acute osteomyelitis in a child.
- Outline the principles of management in case of infected nonunion of long bone. How will you treat infected non-union of tibia?
- Discuss the indications of surgery in TB spine with or without neurological complications.
- Enumerate various diagnostic tests with their relative merits for postoperative infection. Outline the treatment.
- Describe musculoskeletal manifestation of HIV infected patients.
- Describe anatomical classification of chronic osteomyelitis. Discuss the principles of management based on this classification. How will you fill the dead space after excision of infected tissue?
- Enumerate the radiological types of TB hip. How does this classification help in prognosis?
- Rationale for using metallic implants in osteoarticular TB.
- Explain the neurological deficit in caries spine, types, pathogenesis, and prognostic factors.

- Discuss the pathogenesis of acute hematogenous osteomyelitis. How does it differ in age groups?
- What is DOTS? What is its rationale?
- Explain nosocomial infection on orthopedics with its common organisms and preventive measures.
- Describe Madura foot.
- Describe Brodie abscess.

TUMOR

- Describe types and principles of biopsy for musculoskeletal tumor.
- Explain hemophilic cyst.
- Explain musculoskeletal manifestation of neurofibromatosis.
- Explain polyostotic fibrous dysplasia.
- Describe osteitis fibrosa cystica.
- Describe Paget's disease. Explain its clinical features, biochemical investigations, and medical treatment.
- Explain pycnodysostosis.
- Describe Codman's tumor (chondroblastoma).
- Describe chemotherapy for osteosarcoma.
- Describe rotationplasty.
- Describe recent advances in reduction of recurrence in GCT with emphasis on medical treatment.
- Describe extracorporeal RT for bone sarcoma.
- Explain brachytherapy.
- Describe the role of embolization in orthopedics.
- Explain oncogenic osteomalacia.
- Briefly describe the clinical features, types, and management of osteoid osteoma.
- Discuss the pathology, clinical features, and management of synovial chondromatosis.
- Discuss the current concepts in management of osteosarcoma.
- Discuss the current concepts in management of skeletal metastasis.
- Enumerate fibrous lesions of bone. Explain its clinical features, diagnosis, and management of fibrous dysplasia of bone.
- Enumerate principles of limb salvage surgery in malignant bone tumors. List the indications and contraindications. Describe the techniques of limb salvage in osteosarcoma of distal end of femur.
- Differentiate between parosteal and periosteal osteosarcoma in terms of pathology, clinical features, treatment and prognosis.
- Discuss the pathology, clinical features, diagnosis, and treatment of pigmented villonodular synovitis.
- What is "Sandwich technique"? Describe the technique in the management of GCT of distal end of radius.

- Describe clinical features, radiology, and treatment of non-ossifying fibroma.
- Describe clinical presentation, diagnosis and management of multiple myeloma.
- Enumerate the methods to cover defects after excision of primary malignant tumors of bone.
- What is extracorporeal irradiated tumor bone?
- Discuss the pathophysiology, clinical manifestation, and differential diagnosis of heterotopic ossification.
- What is diffuse interstitial skeletal hyperostosis (DISH). Describe the clinical features and its management.
- Describe the pathology, clinical features, radiological findings, and treatment of diaphyseal aclasis (HME).
- What are giant cell variants? Describe in brief their differential diagnosis.
- Explain Campanacci disease (osteofibrous dysplasia).
- Briefly discuss the clinical features and pathology of Ewing's sarcoma. Outline the principles of treatment in a case of Ewing's sarcoma of upper end of humerus.
- Discuss the differential diagnosis of cystic lesions in upper end of humerus in a 10-year-old child. Describe the management of SBC (UBC) in same child.
- Define GCT. Describe in brief clinical features, diagnosis, and management of GCT of upper end tibia.
- Discuss the management of metastasis in spine.
- Discuss role of pamidronate in bone metastasis.
- Discuss brown tumor and synovioma.
- Discuss various methods available for treatment of GCT of proximal tibia in a 30-year-old man.
- Discuss the approach to a patient with suspected bony metastasis with unknown primary tumor.
- Write a short note on PNET.
- Write a short note on round cell tumor.

CONGENITAL/DEVELOPMENTAL ANOMALIES

- Write a short note on metatarsus adductus.
- Write a short note on congenital dislocation of patella.
- Write a short note on tibialization of fibula.
- Explain CTEV: Pirani scoring and Ponseti plaster technique with reference to pathoanatomy.
- Describe angular deformity of knee in children.
- Enumerate various causes of coxa vara.
- Describe the classification, clinical features, and management of tibial hemimelia.

- Discuss the pathoanatomy, radiology, diagnosis, and management of congenital vertical talus.
- Explain cleidocranial dysostosis.
- Explain genu valgum.
- Define torticollis. Enumerate signs and symptoms of congenital torticollis in a 9-year-old child. How will you manage spasmodic torticollis in a child?
- Describe clinical features of osteogenesis imperfecta. Discuss the types of osteogenesis imperfecta. How does it differ from Battered baby syndrome?
- Define congenital muscular torticollis. List the differential diagnosis and management of congenital torticollis.
- Define pseudarthrosis of tibia. Describe its pathogenesis, diagnosis, classification, and management.
- Classify the congenital skeletal limb deficiencies.
- Explain adolescent coxa vara.
- Classify radial club hand. Describe the pathological anatomy and management of a 1-year-old child.
- Classify congenital dislocation of knee. Comment on its differential diagnosis and management.
- What is congenital coxa vara? Describe its pathophysiology and outline principles of management.
- A 1-year-old child has been successfully treated for CTEV. Describe the orthotic management from this time to the completion of treatment.
- Explain Dwyer's osteotomy for CTEV and its indications, steps and complications.
- Explain Sprengel's deformity. Describe its etiopathogenesis, clinical features, and management.
- Describe coxa plana with its clinical and radiological features, differential diagnosis, and principles of treatment.
- Discuss the bowing of tibia in children with its causes, types, and management of congenital bowing.
- Explain congenital postural deformities associated with in utero position.

PEDIATRIC ORTHOPEDICS

- What are the types of epiphysis? Describe various types, methods, and indications of epiphysiodesis.
- Explain the role of USG in DDH.
- Enumerate the differential diagnosis of a limping child (10-year-old). Differentiate between a case of septic arthritis and transient synovitis.
- Discuss the clinical features and management of painful limp with high grade fever in a 5-year-old child.

- Describe post-traumatic physeal bar with its pathology and management.
- Describe etiology and pathoanatomy of DDH. Also explain its clinical and radiological features in diagnosis of DDH. Explain the treatment of unilateral DDH in a 18-month-old child.
- What is pes cavus? Explain etiology, classification of Pes cavus. Discuss Coleman's block test and its interpretation in pes cavus.
- Classify epiphyseal injuries. Describe the treatment principles and complications of each type. What is Langenskiöld procedure?
- Write a short note on cubitus valgus.
- Write a short note on Blount's disease.
- Write a short note on pseudoparalysis of infancy.
- Enumerate the causes of intoeing gait. How will you treat intoeing gait because of hip disorders?
- How will you evaluate a child with genu valgum deformity? Outline the principles of management. What is timed epiphysiodesis?
- Describe the histological zones of growth plate. Discuss the anatomical changes which take place in rickets and SCFE.
- Describe clinical features and pathophysiology of slipped capital femoral epiphysis (SCFE). What could be the medical conditions associated with it? What is the difference in the radiological picture of Delbet type I fracture neck femur and SCFE?
- Classify congenital failure of formation of limbs. Explain Pappas classification for congenital femoral deficiency and management protocol according to Pappas classification.
- Write a short note on Osgood–Schlatter disease.
- Describe the etiopathology, clinical features, and management of SCFE.
- Describe the pathology, clinical features, diagnosis, and treatment of Madelung's deformity.
- Enumerate "Head at Risk sign". Explain prognostic factors and outcome in the treatment of Perthe's disease.
- Define Perthe's disease. Give its classification and describe its clinical features, diagnosis, and management.
- Write a short note on osteochondritis dissecans (OCD).

NEUROMUSCULAR DISORDERS

- Write a short note on diplegia and double hemiplegia.
- What is Gower's sign? Explain clinical findings, investigations, pathology, and treatment with prognosis of Duchenne muscular dystrophy (DMD).
- Write a short note on Becker muscular dystrophy (BMD).
- Write a short note on myositis ossificans.
- Describe the anatomy of iliotibial band and the effects of its contracture on the lower limb (in polio). How did you clinically detect the contracture?

- Describe the etiology, clinical features, and treatment of Sudeck's osteodystrophy.
- Write down the differences between neurogenic and vascular claudication.
- Describe the classification of neurogenic bladder and management.
- Define and classify cerebral palsy. Define crouched gait, its evaluation, and management in a 10-year-old child.
- Explain quadriceps contracture of infancy and childhood.
- Describe the various foot and ankle deformities in cerebral palsy and their management.
- Discuss the principles of rehabilitation of a paraplegic patient.
- Discuss the types of equinus contracture in cerebral palsy and its management.
- Describe the orthotic management of an insensate foot particularly in reference to leprosy.
- Describe the role and mode of action of pharmacological treatment in CP. Explain role of botulinum toxin in CP.
- Discuss the principles of dorsal root rhizotomy in management of static CP.
- Describe the pathoanatomy, clinical features, and management of post-polio calcaneus deformity in a 12-year-old patient.
- What is quadriceps paralysis gait? Discuss its pathomechanics, compensations employed, and corrective measures.
- Enumerate various deformities of foot and ankle seen in post-polio residual paralysis (PPRP). Describe in detail the management of talipes calcaneus.
- What is post-polio equinus deformity of foot? Discuss its etiopathology, evaluation, and management.
- Write a short note on shoulder-hand syndrome.

FRACTURE AND DISLOCATION

- What is Hangman's fracture? Discuss the classification and management of Hangman's fracture.
- Write a short note on Tillaux fracture.
- Explain Malgaigne fracture and clinical signs of fracture pelvis.
- Discuss the management of brachial artery injury in association with supracondylar humerus fracture (pulseless pink hand in supracondylar humerus fracture).
- Write a short note on Battered baby syndrome.
- Discuss the management of non-union of femoral neck fracture with viable head in a 40-year-old patient.
- Discuss the modalities of surgical treatment of distal end radius fracture with their principles.

Question Bank

- Classify fractures of proximal humerus. What is the relevance of blood supply of humeral head in planning management of fracture of proximal humerus? Discuss the management of four part fracture in an elderly man.
- Discuss the principles of wound debridement.
- What is reconstructive ladder for open factures? What is negative wound therapy? And what is fix and close protocol in open fractures?
- What is Hawkin's sign? Describe the blood supply of talus. Classify fracture neck of talus. Discuss their management.
- Classify neglected femoral neck fracture in adults. Treatment with rationale in each type of neglected femoral neck fracture.
- Classify fracture of acetabulum. Discuss the radiographic evaluation and principles of management of acetabulum fracture.
- Write a short note on pseudofracture.
- Write a short note on role of ligamentotaxis in acute trauma.
- Describe sideswipe injuries of elbow. How will you manage such cases?
- Classify trochanteric fractures of hip. Discuss pros and cons of their management with DHS/PFN.
- What are the problems encountered and use of various modalities in surgical management of fragility fracture.
- Classify tibial plateau fracture. What are the mechanism of injury, evaluation, and treatment of each types?
- Discuss acute management of traumatic knee dislocation.
- Write a short note on post-traumatic tibia valga.
- Discuss the mechanism of injury of "Unhappy triad of O'Donoghue".
- Explain the classification of fracture of distal end of radius.
- Classify fracture of calcaneum (Sander's classification) and describe principles of management and complications.
- Describe Hoffa's fracture.
- Describe extensor mechanism of knee. Define the recurrent dislocation of patella. Discuss in brief its clinical features, diagnosis, and treatment.
- Discuss the structure of physis with suitable diagrams. Classify physeal injuries. Describe the management and complications of various types of physeal injuries.
- Enumerate causes of stiff elbow. Discuss the surgical management of post traumatic ankyloses of elbow in extension.
- Classify traumatic dislocation of shoulder. Describe the diagnosis and management of neglected posterior shoulder dislocation in young adult.
- Classify ankle injuries. Discuss in brief the treatment principles of each type.
- Describe blood supply of scaphoid. Describe clinical features, diagnosis, and management of non-union scaphoid.

Question Bank

- Classify fracture neck of femur in children. Discuss the treatment principles and prognosis.
- Describe vascular fibular grafting in the management of neglected fracture neck of femur.
- Describe the Stimson's method to reduce posterior dislocation of hip.
- Classify open fracture of tibia. Describe management of type 3B open fracture of tibia stress fracture.
- Describe the management of fracture shaft humerus with radial nerve palsy. What is Holstein–Lewis lesion and its management?
- Describe the classification of fracture neck of talus. Outline the principles of its management. What is Hawkins Sign?
- Write a short note on labral tears of hip in young athletes.
- Classify pelvic fracture. Describe various radiological views for assessing pelvic injuries. How will you manage rotationally unstable pelvic injuries?
- Classify glenoid fracture and discuss its management. What is floating shoulder and how it is managed?
- Briefly describe the etiology and pathoanatomy of recurrent shoulder dislocation. Outline the principles of management.
- Write a short note on habitual dislocation of patella.
- Describe the clinical presentation of posterior dislocation of hip. How will you reduce it by Bigelow's method? Discuss the causes which make reduction difficult. Enumerate complications of posterior dislocation of hip.
- Write a short note on Torus fracture.
- Discuss the etiology, diagnosis, and management of an infected fracture shaft femur in an adult after surgery for fracture.
- Classify proximal humerus fracture. Explain relevance of blood supply. Discuss management options of various types. Outline the management of type 4 fracture in elderly females.
- Describe the classification of distal humerus fracture in adults. Describe the surgical approaches used for internal fixation of these fracture.
- What are the components of "terrible triad of elbow"? Describe the mechanism and principles of management.
- Define post-traumatic stiff knee. Discuss in brief its cause, diagnosis, and management.
- Classify perioperative femoral stem fracture around hip joint. Discuss the treatment options.
- Describe the classification, clinical features, and management of Lisfranc fracture dislocation.
- Describe the mechanism of injury of radial head fracture. Discuss its classification and management.
- Describe the mechanism of injury and classification of tibial pilon fracture and discuss their management.

- Classify posterior fracture dislocation of femoral head fracture and describe its management.
- Classify fracture of distal end of femur. Discuss the principles of their management.
- Discuss the surgical anatomy of AC joint. Classify AC joint injuries and describe their management.
- Write a short note on stress fracture of neck of femur.
- Write a short note on fracture head of femur.
- Describe classification and management of Monteggia fracture-dislocation.
- Classify distal end radius fracture. Describe radiological indices of wrist. Discuss treatment principles for extra-articular distal radius fracture.
- Define non-union. Describe classification and broad principles of management of diaphyseal non-union.
- Describe briefly the etiology, clinical features, diagnosis, and investigations treatment of painful elbow following injury around elbow.
- What are Monteggia equivalents? Discuss the principles of management of Monteggia fracture dislocation in children.
- What is traumatic arthrotomy of knee joint? What is fluid challenge test to confirm the diagnosis?
- Explain the current concepts in the management of fracture neck and head of radius in children and adults.
- Describe the anatomy of DRUJ. Describe the indications and techniques of performing Kapandji's procedure.
- What is toddler's fracture? Discuss its differential diagnosis and management.
- Classify elbow dislocation. How will you manage an unreduced posterior dislocation elbow in a 10-year-old child?
- What is floating knee? Discuss its management in a 25-year-old adult.
- Discuss the approach to a patient of pelvic fracture with suspected abdominal injury.
- Describe the causes of ulnar wrist pain after healing of distal radial fracture and its management.
- Discuss the advances in the management of periarticular fracture.
- Differentiating features in the pathoanatomy and management of intracapsular neck of femur fracture in children and adults.
- Briefly write management of hemarthrosis of knee developing in an injury.
- Write the indications for valgus osteotomy for fracture neck of femur. Discuss the preoperative planning, implant choice, advantages, and disadvantages of the procedure.
- Classify the capitellum fracture and its management.
- What is LISS? Discuss its role in stabilizing fracture of distal femur.

- Discuss peritalar dislocation and talar fracture.
- What is unstable trochanteric fracture? Briefly describe the methods of managing unstable trochanteric fracture.
- Describe the management of patient having fracture pelvis with urinary retention. Restrict yourself to management of urinary problems.
- Write a short note on Bennett's fracture dislocation.
- Describe fracture disease.
- Write a short note on lateral condyle fracture of humerus.

SPINE

- Discuss the recent advances in management of PID.
- Classify scoliosis. Explain the clinical features and management of idiopathic scoliosis.
- Write a short note on spinal shock.
- What is Brown-Séquard syndrome (BSS)? Explain its etiopathogenesis and clinical features.
- Discuss the spinal cord injury without radiological abnormality (SCIWORA).
- Differentiate between vascular and neurogenic claudication.
- Differentiate between paraplegia with active disease (early onset paraplegia) and healed disease (late onset paraplegia).
- Discuss the "ASIA score". Classify bladder paralysis in spinal cord injury with salient features.
- Define spondylolisthesis. Describe its classification in adults, its clinical features, and radiological signs. Outline its management.
- What is whiplash injury of cervical spine? Discuss its clinical features, diagnosis, and treatment.
- Discuss spinal segment and instability. Explain Canadian C-spine rule and its physiology.
- Discuss pathology, clinical features, diagnosis, and treatment of L4-5 PID.
- Discuss the factors influencing spinal curve progression in congenital scoliosis.
- Describe the anatomy of central and lateral canals in lumber spine in relation to LCS. How will you clinically differentiate central from lateral canal LCS? Briefly describe the management.
- Discuss the principles of application of Milwaukee brace. What are the clinical features of idiopathic kyphoscoliosis. Enumerate the indications of surgical intervention.
- Write a short note on spine at risk sign.
- Discuss the role of injectable methylprednisolone in post-traumatic spinal injury.

- Classify thoracolumbar spine injuries. Give radiological classification of burst fracture. Describe management of L1 burst fracture.
- Describe the mechanism of injury and clinical presentation of various incomplete spinal cord syndromes.
- Describe the pathology, diagnosis, and broad principles of management of ankylosing spondylitis.
- Describe the autonomic dysreflexia in spinal cord injury.
- Describe various types of lumbar root anomalies. List the complication of lumbar disk surgeries.
- Describe endoscopic spinal surgery and its technique.
- What is sacral nutation and its role in chronic low backache?
- What is Klippel–Feil syndrome? Discuss its etiology, pathology, clinical and radiological features, differential diagnosis, and management.
- Describe the pathophysiology and pharmacological treatment of acute spinal cord injury.
- Describe the management of congenital scoliosis.
- Define end vertebrae and apical vertebrae in adolescent idiopathic scoliosis (AIS). Describe two radiological methods to measure the curve in AIS. Explain fusionless technique of correction in idiopathic scoliosis.
- Describe the physiology of micturition. Briefly discuss the management of automatic bladder in spinal injuries.
- What is central cord syndrome? Describe its clinical presentation. How will you manage such cases?
- Discuss sexual and bladder rehabilitation of a 30-year-old male following a complete spinal injury at D12 vertebral level.
- Write a short note on Scheuermann's disease.
- Write a short note on filum terminale syndrome.
- What are the various protocols which have been used for pharmacological intervention in spinal cord injuries? What is the current opinion on pharmacological intervention?
- What are the indications of spinal osteotomy in ankylosing spondylitis? Describe the various techniques.
- Enumerate the types of spinal cord lesions following fracture dislocation of C5-6 vertebrae and discuss clinical features, treatment, and prognosis of each type of lesion in adults.
- Explain pathophysiology of Pott's spine. Describe the routes through which a tubercular abscess can travel to far off regions in the body based on anatomical facts.
- What is the "watershed zone" of the spinal cord? Draw a cross-section of the spinal cord in the dorsal region.
- Describe stages of Pott's paraplegia in a typical paravertebral lesion based on the anatomy of tracts.

SPORTS MEDICINE

- Write a short note on meniscal repair.
- Describe minimal access surgical management of acetabular fracture and its indications, positioning portals and complications of hip arthroscopy.
- Write a short note on autologous chondrocyte implantation.
- Write a short note on platelet rich plasma (PRP).
- Write a short note on painful arc syndrome.
- What are the causes of maltracking of patella?
- Write a short note on triple deformity of knee.
- Describe the scapular dyskinesia and its role in rotator cuff impingement.
- Write a short note on SLAP lesions.
- Classify multiligament knee injury and principles of managing such cases.
- Discuss the increasing role of minimum invasive techniques in orthopedics and role of arthroscopy in management of intra-articular fracture.
- Outline the management of chronic ACL insufficiency in young athlete.
- Write a short note on Bankart lesion.
- Explain frozen shoulder with its clinical features and management.
- Discuss the investigations and management of ACL injury in young athlete reporting after injury.
- Discuss the recent advances in arthroscopic ACL reconstruction with reference to creation of femoral tunnel and femoral fixation methods.
- Describe the anatomy of tibialis posterior tendon. What is posterior tibial tendon dysfunction (PTTD)? Describe the management of such cases.
- Enumerate the portals for arthroscopy of knee joint. Describe the various arthroscopies, their accessories, and indication of arthroscopy of knee joint.
- Write a short note on discoid meniscus.
- Discuss treatment options of the focal cartilage defects over the medial femoral condyle in a 40-year-old man.
- Discuss the diagnosis and management of ACL injury.
- Describe various clinical tests for evaluation of ligamentous injuries of knee.
- Describe role of fibrin gel and chondrocyte culture in orthopedics.
- Define multidisciplinary instability of shoulder joint. Discuss its management.
- Discuss the subacromial impingement syndrome.
- What do you understand by patellar instability? Describe the principles of management, before and after skeletal maturity.

- Discuss anatomy of rotator cuff. What is rotator cuff disease?
- Describe various clinical methods to diagnose ACL injury. Describe postoperative management of ACL reconstruction by bone patellar tendon bone graft.
- Enumerate various methods of ACL reconstruction. Discuss the pros and cons of each method.
- Explain loose bodies in knee. Describe its etiology and classification. How will you manage a case of a 30-year-old sportsman who presents with locked knee due to loose body?
- Describe anatomy of subacromial space. What is the morphology of acromion process in the pathogenesis of rotator cuff tears? How will you manage full-thickness tear?
- Discuss current status of hip arthroscopy. Explain its indications in contemporary orthopedic practice and explain the important steps of the procedure.

NERVE INJURIES

- Explain the classification and electrodiagnostic studies of nerve injuries.
- Explain the course of radial nerve and its applied surgical significance.
- Write a short note on motor march.
- Classify nerve injuries. Describe pathology of nerve regeneration, methods of nerve repair and methods of closing gaps between nerve ends.
- Write a short note on tendon transfer for ulnar nerve palsy.
- Write a short note on Wallerian degeneration.
- Describe the principles of tendon transfer. Discuss the tendon transfer for high radial nerve palsy (modified Jones transfer).
- Describe the anatomy of common peroneal nerve. Name the muscles supplied by the nerve and the tendon transfers in CPN palsy.
- Draw a labeled diagram of brachial plexus. Classify brachial plexus injury. Describe clinical features and management of lower brachial plexus injury.
- Discuss the management of claw hand in a patient suffering from leprosy.
- Describe the AIN syndrome. Explain its etiology, clinical features, differential diagnosis, and management.
- Write a short note on Erb's palsy.
- Discuss the management of closed fracture of shaft of humerus with radial nerve palsy.
- Describe the surgical reconstruction in a case of one and half year old CPN palsy.
- Draw a cross-section of peripheral nerve and label its structures.
- Describe the early tendon transfer in radial nerve palsy.

- Define ulnar claw hand. Enumerate the causes of ulnar claw hand. Discuss its management.
- Describe pathophysiology of nerve compression (entrapment) syndrome. Enumerate various syndromes of nerve entrapment.
- Describe methods of closing gaps between nerve ends during nerve repair.
- Enumerate expendable nerves and explain about donor site morbidity of common donor nerves.
- Discuss orthotic management in high radial nerve palsy.
- Discuss clinical differentiation between preganglionic and post-ganglionic lesions of brachial plexus and its effect on management.
- What is neuropraxia? How will you differentiate it from axonotmesis during first few days of injury?
- Name the prehensile movements of hand. What are the tendon transfers described for opponens deficit hand?
- What is crutch palsy? Describe orthotic management of wrist drop.

MICROSURGERY

- Describe the principles of coverage of soft tissue defect and bone gap in tibia in mid leg in a patient with feeble distal pulses.
- Discuss the prevention and treatment of pressure sores and UTI in paraplegic patients.
- Write a short note on induced membrane formation to cover bone defects.
- Describe the gluteus maximus flap in the management of decubitus ulcer.
- Describe free vascularized bone transplant. Describe the principles of techniques and application in orthopedic practice.
- What is flap reconstruction? Write its classification.
- How will you transport an organ after amputation in sterilized center for reimplantation? What is the order of implantation in a below elbow amputation?
- Describe the various myocutaneous flaps used to cover tibia in different levels.
- Describe various types of skin grafts. Discuss the stages of biological incorporation of skin grafts.

HAND AND WRIST

- What is Kanavel's sign? Describe management of suppurative flexor tenosynovitis of hand.
- Write a short note on intrinsic plus hand.
- Write a short note on ulnar paradox.

- Describe Dupuytren's disease and its characteristic features. Describe in brief its pathogenesis, prognosis, and management.
- Explain flexor zones of hand. Describe clinical features and management of a 2-month-old with zone 2 injury.
- Define carpal tunnel syndrome. Describe pathological anatomy, causes, diagnosis, and management of carpal tunnel syndrome.
- Outline the treatment of flexor tendon injury (acute and chronic) in zone 2.
- Describe the potential spaces of hand. Discuss clinical features and treatment of deep space infection of hand.
- What is felon? What is its preferred management? How it is different from paronychia?
- Write a short note on compound palmar ganglion.
- Define trigger finger. Enumerate causes of trigger finger. Describe the clinical picture and surgical treatment of trigger thumb.
- What is Dupuytren's fracture-dislocation? Discuss its management.
- Write a short note on mallet finger.
- Describe the anatomy of FDS and FDP in hand.
- Describe tendon repair techniques and important suture configurations.
- Enumerate various causes of claw hand. What is the pathogenesis of clawing? Discuss the principles of surgical correction.
- Describe instability pattern after wrist trauma. Discuss the management of VISI (volar intercalated segment instability).
- Classify flexor tendon injuries of hand. Describe the treatment of neglected ruptures of flexor tendon in zone 2.
- Describe various functions of hand. How will you attain key pinch in a quadriplegic with no useful power?
- Describe carpal instability and its types, clinical features and radiological assessment.
- Describe the pathoanatomy of bursae of the hand. Discuss the etiology, clinical features, and management of acute infection in those bursae.
- Write a short note on perilunar dislocation.
- Describe pollicization and its indications and prerequisites.

FOOT AND ANKLE

- Write a short note on foot drop and equinus deformity.
- Enumerate causes, pathoanatomy and clinical features of TA rupture and treatment of a fresh rupture.
- Describe tarsal tunnel syndrome and its clinical features and management.
- Describe the principles of stabilization of foot.
- Describe in brief etiology, pathology, clinical features, and principles of management of Charcot joint (diabetic foot).

- Describe muscular dynamics in calcaneovalgus deformity. Describe management in patients before and after attaining skeletal maturity.
- Describe the pathogenesis of hallux valgus deformity. Describe the role of metatarsus primary varus in pathogenesis. How will you manage an adolescent girl with severe hallux valgus?
- Discuss the indications, merits, and demerits of talectomy.
- Describe the arches of foot. Classify flat foot briefly and discuss the management principles of flat feet in child.

HIP AND PELVIS

- Describe the stage of TB arthritis of hip. Differentiating clinical features, treatment, and prognosis of each stage.
- Enumerate causes of AVN of femoral head and nonarthroplasty surgical management of AVN of femoral head. Describe core decompression.
- Describe the blood supply of femoral head. How does it differ in children and adults?
- Why a patient with hip pain walks with a stick in the opposite hand? Illustrate your answer with suitable diagrams.
- Write a short note on femoroacetabular impingement syndrome.
- Describe Salter's osteotomy. What are its indications, principle technical steps, merits, and demerits?
- Classify AVN. Enumerate pathology and outline the principles of management of Ficat
- Enumerate stage 3 AVN of femoral head in a 30-year-old man.
- What is pelvic support osteotomy? Outline its principles and operative technique.
- What are anatomical and physiological difference between neck shaft angle and version in child and adults?
- Define femoral anteversion. How do you detect it clinically? Discuss the role of anteversion in orthopedic diagnosis and management.
- Write a short note on otto pelvis (protrusio acetabuli).

ARTHROPATHY AND INFLAMMATORY DISORDERS

- Describe with the diagram of extensor expansion of finger. Explain pathological anatomy of boutonniere and swan-neck deformities in RA.
- Write a short note on biological agents used in treatment of RA.
- Write a short note on morning stiffness.
- Write a short note on the role of DMARD in RA.
- Differentiate between RA and OA.
- Describe recent advances in diagnosis and management of RA.
- Define gout. Describe in brief its clinical features, diagnosis, and treatment.

- Define and enumerate the etiology of neuropathic arthropathy. Discuss in brief its diagnosis and principles of management.
- Discuss the pathology of OA knee with special reference to the role of ACL rupture in pathogenesis of OA knee.
- Write a short note on allopurinol.
- Write a short note on sacroiliitis with its etiology and diagnosis

INVESTIGATIONS AND CLINICAL TESTS

- Draw a diagram of strength duration curve and write about its clinical significance.
- Write a short note on PET scan.
- Explain the application of MRI in diagnosis and management of spinal tumors.
- Explain nuclear medicine and role of nuclear scan in orthopedics.
- Write a short note on whole body CT scan in trauma.
- Write a short note on nerve conduction velocity.
- Write a short note on bone scan.
- Explain the principles of ultrasonography. Discuss its clinical use in orthopedics.
- Write a short note on electromyography.
- Write a short note on electrodiagnosis in carpal tunnel syndrome.
- Describe Trendelenburg test with its anatomical basis and clinical application.
- Write a short note on electrodiagnostic studies.
- Write a short note on role of ultrasound in fracture healing.
- Explain the role of labeled WBC and multiphasic bone scan in bone pathology.
- Write a short note on Ober's test and modified Ober's test.

ORTHOTICS AND PROSTHESIS

- Expandable megaprosthesis.
- Describe Jaipur foot and differentiate between SACH foot and Jaipur foot.
- Write a short note on bionic hand.
- Write a short note on Knuckle Bender Splint.
- Write a short note on PTB cast.
- What is myoelectric prosthesis? Describe its components, applications, and advantages.
- Write a short note on Halo-pelvic device.
- Write a short note on Steenbeck brace.
- Draw a diagram of floor reaction orthosis. Describe indications and contraindications for its use. Describe its mechanism of action.

- Describe the role of orthosis in treatment of club foot.
- Describe PTB prosthesis and its indications, prerequisites and advantages.
- Describe Pavlik harness.
- Describe SOMI brace.
- Describe Jaipur Foot. Discuss the difference between SACH foot and Madras foot.
- Discuss the principles of application of functional cast bracing in the management of diaphyseal fracture of long bones.
- Write a short note on thermoplastic splints.
- Define ankle foot orthosis. What are the plastic materials used in fabrication? Describe indications and care during daily use.
- Write a short note on hanging cast.
- Discuss suction socket prosthesis and its principles, indications and advantages over conventional prosthesis and main points in its construction.
- Describe various types of crutches and gait pattern with crutches.
- What are the parts of a shoe? Describe the modification of a CTEV shoe.

IMPLANTS AND SURGICAL TECHNIQUES

- What are the attachments of GT? Describe indications and steps of safe surgical dislocation of hip.
- Discuss the types of frames and methods to increase the stability of external fixator. How will you prevent complications of external fixator?
- Explain Surgical steps of Hardinge approach of hip.
- Discuss the tension band principles. Describe its clinical use in fracture management.
- Write a short note on wake-up test.
- Write a short note on MIPPO.
- Write a short note on fracture fixation using shape memory (NINITOL) staples.
- Write a short note on tension band plating
- Explain principles of management of intercondylar fracture humerus and Bryan–Morrey approach (triceps reflecting approach).
- Explain surgical anatomy of Ganz approach to hip joint.
- Discuss modified Stoppa approach for acetabulum fractures.
- Discuss evolution of plate osteosynthesis starting from "Sherman" plates to present day locking plates. What are the principles of locking plate osteosynthesis including their advantages and disadvantages?
- What are biodegradable implants? What is their chemical composition? Mention the indications of their use, advantages, and disadvantages.
- Discuss surgical steps of anterolateral decompression D5-6 spine.
- Write a short note on Herbert screw.
- Write a short note on skeletal traction in acute trauma.

- Write a short note on surgical steps of anterolateral exposure of hip.
- List the osteotomies around hip. Write briefly about the principles of each osteotomy.
- Advances in articular cartilage tissue engineering.
- What are the commonly used orthopedic sutures in orthopedics? Compare their properties.
- Describe Ilizarov fixator and corticotomy. How will you manage a case of defect nonunion?
- Write a short note on bikini incision.
- Write a short note on Schanz osteotomy.
- What is bone cement? What are the indications and CI for its use? What are the methods of cementing techniques? Discuss their differences in brief.
- Write down indications of hip arthrography. Discuss various approaches to aspirate hip joint.
- Write a short note on valgus osteotomy.
- Explain the effects of reaming of bone.
- What are the indications of excision of head of radius? Describe the posterolateral approach.
- Describe principles, merits, and pitfalls in using LCP.
- Describe the design of pelvic "C" clamp. What are the indications of its application and method to fix an unstable pelvic fracture?
- Write a short note on plaster of Paris.
- Describe with illustrative diagrams the surgical exposures of radius at various levels.
- Describe stress, strain and Young's modulus of elasticity in relation to orthopedic implants.
- Describe briefly the approach to hip. Mention advantages and disadvantages of each approach.
- Differentiate between machine screw and ASIF screw.
- Write short notes on: DCP, LCDCP, and LCP.
- Write a short note on Perrins hypothesis.
- Differentiate between static compression and dynamic compression.
- Explain osteochondral allograft transplantation. Mention indications for the procedure.
- Explain Ganz antishock pelvic fixator.
- Explain malalignment test. Discuss the principles of focal dome osteotomy.
- Elaborate the principles of LCP. What are the applications in periarticular fracture?
- Explain trochanteric flip osteotomy in surgical exposure of hip joint.
- Describe various systems, implants available for limb length equalization.
- Discuss their underlying principles.

- Explain the principles and biomechanics of IM nailing.
- Explain the principles of chondroplasty in OA knee.
- Discuss the indications, pros and cons of reamed versus unreamed IM nailing.
- Write a short note on Bryant's traction.
- Write a short note on Harmon's approach of tibia with applied anatomy.
- Explain Chiari osteotomy and its indications, advantages, and steps of surgery.

PHYSIOTHERAPY

- Write a short note on interferential therapy (IFT).
- Write a short note on isokinetic exercises.
- What is isotonic contraction? Classify isotonic muscle contraction.
- What is SWD? How is it different from microwave diathermy. Discuss indications and CI of SWD and microwave diathermy.
- What are closed chain and open chain exercises and discuss ACL rehabilitation protocol?
- What are the various types of exercises? Discuss the benefits and indications of isometric exercises.
- Write a short note on transcutaneous electric nerve stimulation (TENS).
- What is paraffin wax? How is it useful in treatment of orthopedic conditions. What are the indications and contraindications of wax bath therapy?
- Explain ultrasonic therapy and its physiological effects, clinical applications and contraindications.
- Write a short note on cryotherapy
- Write a short note on LASER and its applications in orthopedics.
- Discuss microwave diathermy and its physiological effects, clinical applications, and contraindications.

METABOLIC DISORDERS

- Discuss clinical presentation and management of senile osteoporosis.
- Describe the pathology and radiological signs in rickets and scurvy.
- Explain role of bisphosphonates in the management of osteoporosis and their complications.
- Discuss the mechanism of action of teriparatide in treatment of osteoporosis and potential complication of teriparatide.
- Write a short note on fluorosis.
- Write a short note on Albers-Schönberg disease.
- Define peak bone mass. What factors affect attaining peak bone mass? How does it correlate with osteoporosis?

- Define and classify osteoporosis. Explain radiological investigations in a patient with osteoporosis. How will you manage a case of fracture D12 in an adult?
- Discuss the etiopathogenesis, clinical features, and management of alkaptonuria (ochronotic arthropathy).
- Differentiate between osteonecrosis and transient migratory osteoporosis.
- Outline the calcium metabolism. What do you mean by vitamin D resistant rickets? Describe its clinical features and management.
- Enumerate various methods for bone mineral measurements. Define its density in various conditions.
- Explain effect of chronic kidney disease on bone.
- Write a short note on juvenile idiopathic osteoporosis.
- Discuss anatomy of parathyroid gland. Discuss role of PTH in calcium metabolism and clinical features and radiological presentation of adenoma of parathyroid. What is hungry bone syndrome?
- Describe the etiology, clinical features, diagnosis, and treatment of renal osteodystrophy.
- Describe bony changes in hyperparathyroidism and hypoparathyroidism along with relevant physiology.
- Define and classify rickets. Describe pathogenesis, clinical features, and management of hypophosphatemic rickets.
- What is the indication and principles of behind PTH therapy for treatment of osteoporosis. What are its merits and demerits?
- Write a short note on osteomalacia.
- Write a short note on crystal synovitis.

PSM

- Write a short note on randomized control trial.
- What is evidence-based medicine. Define the hierarchy of evidence and broad principles of each type. Discuss the differences in various types of studies
- Write a short note on plagiarism.
- Write a short note on impact factor.
- Write a short note on telemedicine.
- Draw a flowchart of disaster planning at state level. What is the concept of triage?

MISCELLANEOUS

- Write a short note on nanotechnology
- Write a short note on medical ethics in orthopedics.
- Define component therapy. Enumerate and uses of various blood fractions.

- What is cast syndrome? Enumerate its clinical symptoms and discuss its management.
- Write a short note on methotrexate in orthopedics.
- Write a short note on chymopapain.
- Write a short note on SPONK (spontaneous osteonecrosis of knee).
- Explain schwannoma and its clinical features and diagnosis.
- Describe calculation of CORA and explain with diagram.
- Write a short note on Ehlers–Danlos syndrome.
- Explain the role of botulinum neurotoxin in orthopedic surgery.
- Write a short note on alendronate-induced fracture.
- Write a short note on sexual dimorphism in orthopedic practice.
- What is Marfan syndrome? What is its orthopedic management?
- How will you manage a case of recalcitrant tennis elbow?
- Write a short note on control of air quality in modern orthopedic OT.
- Write a short note on Raloxifene.
- Write a short note on Milwaukee shoulder syndrome.
- Write a short note on 3D C-arm.
- Write a short note on EUSOL.
- Describe interventional radiology in orthopedics. Write two examples.
- Describe the principles of gamma camera (γ-camera) and radioactive substance(s) used in gamma camera. Discuss indications and use of gamma camera.
- Describe intravenous regional anesthesia in orthopedic practice.
- Write a short note on day-care surgery.
- Write a short note on surgical audit.

Index

A

Acetabular depth 124
Acetabular index 124
Acetabular version 125
Acetabulum fracture 18
Achterman and Kalamchi classification 89
Acromioclavicular joint 115
    injuries 3
Adult respiratory distress syndrome 110
Aitken's classification 84
Allen classification 15
Allman classification 1
Alpha and beta angles 65
Anal atresia 81
Anatomical axis 127
Anderson and d'Alonzo classification 47
Anderson and Montesano classification 45
Ankle 132
    fractures 30
Ankylosing spondylitis 106
Anomalies, congenital 78
AO classification 29
Apert syndrome 82
Aplasia, partial 83
Arc
    first 14
    greater 13
    lesser 13
    second 14
    third 14
Arnold and Hilgartner classification, modified 104
Arthritis 107
Arthroscopic classification 54
Arthroscopic staging 51
Atlantoaxial rotatory subluxation and dislocation 47
Atlanto-occipital dislocation 46
Atlas fracture 46
Avascular necrosis 65

B

Bado classification 9
Bateman classification 54
Baumann's angle 117
Baumgartner index 111

Beighton criteria 110
Bending injury 11
Berndt and Harty classification 70
Best motor response 93
Best verbal response 94
Bimastoid line 139
Bipartite patella 69
Blackburne-Peel index 131
Blauth classification 82
Blount's disease 84
Blumensaat's line 129
Bohler's angle 133
Bone
    destruction, pattern of 101
    forearm fracture, both 42
Boyd and Griffin classification 23
Boyd and Knight classification 34
Boyd classification 85
Brachial plexus injury 53
Brain injury 94
Breathing, increased 110
Burst fracture 47

C

Calcaneus fracture 35
Calcific tendinitis 51
Cam impingement 67
Campanacci classification 100
Cardiac defects 81
Carrying angle 118
Caton-Deschamps index 130
Catterall classification 59
Cavendish classification 78
Center-edge angle 125
Central stenosis 73
Cervical spine 136-139
Chamberlain line 138
Charcot's arthropathy 71
Checketts-Otterburn grading 99
Cheng's clinical group 79
Choi's classification 99
Chondromalacia patella 68
Chopart fracture 36
Cierny-Mader classification 96
Clavicle fracture 1
Cobb angle, indirect 141
Cobb method 140, 141

Cofield classification 54
Condyle humerus physeal fractures,
    lateral 41
Contralateral hip 125
Coronoid fracture 7
Crawford classification 86
C-reactive protein 106
Crowe classification 63
Crude memorization technique 32
Cuff tears, complete 54
Cuff, width of 113

D

Dameron-Lawrence-Bofte classification 37
Danis-Weber classification 32
de Carvalho index 131
de Lee classification 37
Degenerative spondylolisthesis 75
Degenerative triangular fibrocartilage
    complex tears, classification of 15
Delbet classification 43
Denis classification 50
Diabetic foot 71
Diffuse idiopathic skeletal hyperostosis 108
Diffuse osteomyelitis 97
Digastric line 140
Dimeglio scoring 87
Disk
    degeneration 76
    extrusion 75, 76
    prolapse 75, 76
    protrusion 75, 76
    sequestration 75, 76
Displacement, direction of 55
Distal femur fracture 25
Distal radioulnar joint 15
Distal radius fracture 11
Doyle classification 15
Dupuytren's contracture 53
Dysplastic spondylolisthesis 75

E

Eastwood classification 53
Eichenholtz classification 71
Elbow 116
    dislocation 7
    heterotopic ossification of 103
    instability 55
    shaft condylar angle 118
Elementary fracture 18
Elephant foot 94
Elizabethtown classification 62
Ellis classification, modified 29
End-organ damage 109

Enneking classification 99
Enthesitis-related arthritis 107
Epstein classification 21
Erythrocyte sedimentation rate 106
Essex-Lopresti classification 35
Evans classification 23
Extraforaminal stenosis 73
Eye opening 94
Eyre-Brook classification 97

F

Fat embolism 109
Fat pad sign 116
Felix classification 102
Femoral shaft fractures 25
Femoroacetabular impingement 67
Femur 102
    fracture
        head of 21
        neck of 22
        neglected neck of 22
    ipsilateral fractures of 28
    neck nonunion 96
Fernandez classification 11
Fibula, hypoplasia of 89
Fibular hemimelia 89
Ficat and Arlet classification 65
Fielding and Hawkins classification 47
Fielding classification 24
Final deformity, calculation of 114
Fingertip injuries 15
Flexibility index 114
Flexor tenosynovitis, criteria for 105
Floating knee 28
Foot 135
    and ankle fractures 30
    intermetatarsal angle of 135
    kite's angle, of 136
Foraminal stenosis 73
Fracture
    burst 47
    description 101
    dislocations 13
    elementary 18
    lateral mass 47
    navicular 36
    of distal segment 1
    of middle third 1
    of proximal third 2
    open 90
    posterior arch 46
    radius 12
    sacral 50
    simple 18
    types of 46

Frankel classification, modified 45
Fraser classification 28
Frykman classification 12

G

Gait 91
Galeazzi fracture 11
Ganga diabetic foot classification 71
Ganga Hospital Scoring System 92
Ganz subtypes 67
Garden classification 22
Gartland classification 40
Giant cell tumor 100
Gibbus deformity 75
Gilula's arc 120
Gilula's lines 14
Gissane's angle 134
Glasgow Coma Scale 93
Glenohumeral dislocation 5
Gothic arch 115
Graham's criteria 123
Griffith Seddon classification 77
Gunshot wound 91
Gurd and Wilson's criteria 109
Gustilo-Anderson classification 90

H

Hallux interphalangeal angle 135
Hallux valgus 70
    angle 135
Hamanishi classification 88
Hand anomalies, congenital 80
Hangman's fracture 48
Hasting and Grahams classification 103
Hawkins classification 34
Head sphericity 125
Heikel classification 81
Hemitransverse
    anterior 20
    posterior 20
Hemophilia 104
Herbert classification 12
Hereditary multiple exostoses 100
Herring lateral pillar classification 60
Hilgenreiner epiphyseal angle 126
Hilgenreiner line 126
Hindfoot contracture score 87
Hip 123
    biomechanics of 111
    developmental dysplasia of 63
    dislocation 20
    periprosthetic fracture of 101
    ultrasound of affected 65
Hohl-Moore classification 28

Horse hoof 94
Humeral and radiocapitellar lines, X-ray
    anterior 117
Humeral line, anterior 116
Hunka classification 97
Hyperlaxity 110
Hypoplasia 83
Hypoplastic radius 81

I

Ideberg classification 2
Ilioischial line 123
Iliopectineal line 123
Iliopubic line 123
Ilium 123
Ilizarov lengthening 112
Impaction injury 11
Impingement syndrome 51
Infraclavicular lesion 54
Injury severity score 92
Insall-Salvati index 113, 129
Insertional tendinitis 72
Intercondylar humerus fracture 6
Intermetatarsal angle, first-second 135
Intertrochanteric fractures 23
Intervertebral disk prolapse 75
Intra-articular fractures 16
    glenoid 2
Isthmic spondylolisthesis 75

J

Jakob classification 41
Jefferson's fracture 46, 47
Jersey finger 16
Johnson and Strom classification 72
Jones, Barnes, Lloyd-Roberts
    classification 88
Juvenile rheumatoid arthritis 107

K

Kalamchi classification 84
Kanavel's sign 105
Kellgren and Lawrence classification 67
Kidner classification 69
Kienbock's disease 57
Kite's angle 136
Klein's line 126
Knee 128
    dislocation 28
Kocher criteria 105
Kumar's clinicoradiological
    classification 77

Kuwada algorithm 72
Kyphosis 75
    congenital 75
    mild 77
    moderate 77
    severe 77

L

Langenskiold classification 84
Lauge-Hansen classification 30
Leddy classification 16
Leighton classification 96
Letournel and Judet classification 18
Letts' classification 11
Levine and Edwards classification 46, 48
Lewis and Rorabeck classification 102
Lichtman classification 57
Limb
    abnormalities 81
    ischemia 91
    length discrepancy 103, 112
Lindeque criteria 109
Lisch nodules 108
Lisfranc fracture 35
Looser classification 104
Lower limb 113
    regional conditions 59
    scanogram of bilateral 128
    trauma 17
Lumbar canal stenosis 73
    anatomic classification 73

M

Maculé-Beneyto classification 11
Madelung deformity 83
Main and Jowett classification 36
Mallet finger 15
Mangled Extremity Severity Score 91
Mann's classification 70
Masada classification 100
Mason classification 9
Mass fracture, lateral 47
Mast and Pappas classification 33
Matsen's classification 5
Mayfield classification 57
Mayo classification 8
McAfee classification 49
McGregor line 138
McRae line 139
Meary's angle
    anteroposterior 135
    lateral 135

Mechanical axis 127
Medial condyle humerus physeal
    fractures 41
Medullary osteomyelitis 97
Mehne and Matta classification 6
Menelaus method 112
Metaphyseal blanch sign 127
Metaphyseal-diaphyseal angle 118
Metatarsal fracture 37
Meyerding's classification 73
Midfoot contracture score 87
Milch classification 41
Mirels' criteria 107
Monteggia equivalents 10
Monteggia fracture 9
    pediatric 11
Morrey and Peterson's criteria 105
Motor vehicle accident 91
Muller AO classification 25
Multiple myeloma 109
Musculotendinous and nerve units 93
Myerson algorithm 72
Myerson classification 36

N

Nail size, calculation of 112
Neck of femur, fractures of 43
Neck shaft angle 125
Neer classification 3
Neer-Horowitz classification 39
Nervous system tumors 79
Neurofibromatosis 108
Neurogenic origin 78
Noninsertional tendinitis 72
Nonosseous 79
Nonunion 94
Nutritional kyphosis 75

O

O'brien classification 42
O'driscoll classification 55
Occipital condyle fracture 45
Odontoid process, fractures of 47
Ogden modification 39
Olecranon fracture 8
Oligoarthritis 107
Orthopedics, formulas in 111
Osseous 79
    classification 67
    origin 78
Osteoarthritis 67
Osteochondritis dissecans 70

Osteogenesis imperfecta 104
Osteomyelitis 96
    diagnosing 105
    localized 97
    superficial 97
Osteotomy
    change in length after 112
    wedge 111
Outerbridge classification 68

P

Paley classification 95
Paraplegia
    early-onset 77
    late-onset 77
Patella
    alta 129
    baja 129
    fracture classification 26
Pathologic spondylolisthesis 75
Pauwel's classification 22
Pediatric trauma 38
Peltola and Vahvanen's criteria 105
Pelvic
    fracture 17
        pediatric 43
    incidence 146
    slope angle 145
    tilt 145
        angle 146
Pelvis
    false 123
    ilioischial line 124
    iliopectineal line 124
    iliopubic line 124
    true 123
Percentage slip calculation 143
Perilunate dislocation 13, 57
Perilunate instability 120
Periprosthetic fracture around knee 102
Periprosthetic infection 103
Perkin's line 125
Perthes disease 59
Peterson type fracture 38
Physiologic host 96
Piece-of-pie sign 120
Pin tract site infection 99
Pincer impingement 67
Pipkin classification 21
Pirani scoring 87
Plexiform neurofibroma 108
Plumb line 140, 144
Polyarthritis 107

Post-traumatic kyphosis 75
Postural kyphosis 75
Powers ratio 137
Pronation external rotation 31
Proximal and distal rows 120
Proximal femoral focal deficiency 84
Proximal humerus fracture 3, 39
Proximal tibial fractures 27
Psoriatic arthritis 107
Pubis 123

Q

Quadriceps angle 128
Quenu and Kuss classification 35

R

Radial bow calculation 113
Radial club hand 81
Radial head
    and neck fractures 42
    classification 9
Radial height 121
    and ulnar variance 122
Radial inclination 121
Radiocapitellar line 117
Radiological lines 115
Radioulnar synostosis, congenital 79
Radius, partial absence of 81
Recess stenosis, lateral 73
Recurrent shoulder dislocation 5
Reflex sympathetic dystrophy 58
Regan and Morrey classification 7
Renal abnormalities 81
Resnick and Niwayama criteria 108
Respiratory failure 110
Respiratory symptoms 110
Retropharyngeal space 137
Rheumatism classification 106
Rheumatoid arthritis 106
    functional classification of 103
Rheumatoid factor 106
Rib vertebral angle difference 142
Ring constriction syndrome 83
Riseborough and Radin classification 6
Risser sign 126
Rockwood classification 3
Rolando and Bennett fracture 16
Rome's criteria 106
Rotator cuff tears 54
    partial thickness 54
Ruedi and Allgower classification 33
Russell-Taylor classification 24

S

Sacral slope 145
Sagittal balance 144
Salter-Harris
　classification 39
　fracture 41
　physeal injury 38
Salter-Thompson classification 59
Sanders classification 35
Sandhu's classification 22
Sangeorzan's classification 36
Saupe classification 69
Scaphoid fracture 12
Scaphoid lunate advanced collapse 56
Scapholunate dissociation 120
Scapula
　fractures 2
　winging of 78
Schams sign 126
Schatzker classification 27
Schenck classification 28
Scheuermann's kyphosis 75
Schöttle's point 129
Scoliosis 114
　and plumb line 141
　positive 141
Scottish terrier sign 143
Seinsheimer classification 25
Septic arthritis
　acute 105
　sequelae 97
Serology 106
Shaft condylar angle 118
Shapiro classification 103, 104
Shear injury 11
Shenton's angle 124
Shenton's line 123
Shock 91
Short distal radius 81
Shoulder 115
Sillence classification 104
Singh index 127
Skeletal structures 93
　bone and joints 93
Skeletal tissue injury 91
Slip angle 144
　calculation 144
Slip, percentage of 143
Slipped capital femoral epiphysis 63
Snyder classification 52
Soft-tissue
　injury 91
　origin 78
Spilled teacup sign 121

Spinal cord injury 45
Spinal disorders 73
Spinal tuberculosis 76
　anatomical involvement 76
Spine 136
　at risk 107
　instability 108
　trauma 45
Spondylolisthesis 73
Spondyloptosis 73
Spoon hand 83
Sprengel's shoulder 78
Steinberg classification 66
Stulberg classification 61
Subtrochanteric femur fractures 24
Sulcus angle 131
Superior labrum
　anterior tear 52
　posterior tear 52
Supination external rotation 30
Supination-adduction 30
Supracondylar elbow fracture 40
Swanson classification 80, 83
Syndactyly 82
Systemic arthritis 107

T

Talar body fracture 34
Talar neck fractures 34
Talar shift 133
Talar tilt 132
Talipes equinovarus, congenital 87
Talocalcaneal angle 136
Talocrural angle 132
Talus 70
Tear drop 119, 123, 124
Tendo Achilles
　chronic injury classification 72
　disorders 72
Terry Thomas sign 120
Thompson and Epstein classification 20
Thoracolumbar fractures 49
Thoracolumbar injury classification 49
Thoracolumbar scoliosis 141
Thumb
　anomaly types 81
　fractures of base of 16
　hypoplasia of 82
Tibia 102
　congenital pseudarthrosis of 85
　hemimelia 88
　ipsilateral fractures of 28
　vara, congenital 84

Tibial fractures 29
Tibial pilon fracture 33
Tibial tubercle fractures 44
Tibial tuberosity 132
  index 113
Tibialis posterior insufficiency 72
Tibiocalcaneal angle 133
Tibiofemoral alignment 129
Tibiofibular clear space 132
Tibiofibular overlap 132
Tibiofibular shaft fractures 29
Tibiotalar angle 134
Tile classification 17
Tip-apex distance 111
Tissues, functional 93
Tönnis angle 124
Torg ratio 137
Torode and Zieg classification 43
Torsion wedge 95
Torticollis 79
Tourniquet pressure 113
Trabecular alignment,
  displacement of 22
Tracheal-esophageal abnormalities 81
Traumatic spondylolisthesis 48, 75
Traumatic triangular fibrocartilage
  complex injuries, classification
  of 14
Traynelis classification 46
Trethowan sign 126
Triangular fibrocartilage injuries 14
Trigger finger 53
Triphalangism 80
Trochlear dysplasia 131
Tscherne classification 90
Tsukayama classification 103
TT:TG distance 132
Tuberculosis spine 114
  paraplegia 76, 77
Tuli staging of 76
Tumor, malignant 99

U

Ulna, bowed 81
Ulnar club hand 83
Ulnar styloid fracture 12
Ulnar variance 122
Ultrasound classification system, Graf
  method for 64
Umbilical artery, single 81
Upper limb 113
  regional conditions 51
  trauma 1

V

Valgus posterolateral rotatory 55
Vancouver classification 101
Vender and Watson classification 83
Vertebral abnormalities 81
Vertical talus, congenital 88
Volar inclination 122
Volar tilt 122

W

Wackenheim line 139
Wagner classification 71
Waldenström sign 125
Watson and Jones classification 44
Watson classification 56
Weber classification 94
White and Panjabi criteria 108
Wilkins classification 42
Wiltse-Newman classification 75
Winquist and Hansen classification 25
Wrist 119
Wynne-Davies criteria 110

Y

Young-Burgess classification 18